Key Facts in
Gastroenterology

TOPICS IN GASTROENTEROLOGY

Series Editor: **Howard M. Spiro, M.D.**
Yale University School of Medicine

COLON
Structure and Function
Edited by Luis Bustos-Fernandez, M.D.

KEY FACTS IN GASTROENTEROLOGY
Jonathan Halevy, M.D.

MEDICAL ASPECTS OF DIETARY FIBER
Edited by Gene A. Spiller, Ph.D., and Ruth McPherson Kay, Ph.D.

MODERN CONCEPTS IN GASTROENTEROLOGY
Edited by Alan B. R. Thomson, M.D., L. R. DaCosta, M.D., and William C. Watson, M.D.

NUTRITION AND DIET THERAPY
IN GASTROINTESTINAL DISEASE
Martin H. Floch, M.D.

PANCREATITIS
Peter A. Banks, M.D.

A Continuation Order Plan is available for this series. A continuation order will bring delivery of each new volume immediately upon publication. Volumes are billed only upon actual shipment. For further information please contact the publisher.

Key Facts in Gastroenterology

Jonathan Halevy, M.D.

Tel Aviv University
Tel Aviv, Israel
and Beilinson Medical Center
Petah Tiqva, Israel

Plenum Medical Book Company • New York and London

Library of Congress Cataloging in Publication Data

Halevy, Jonathan.
  Key facts in gastroenterology.

  (Topics in gastroenterology)
  Includes bibliographies and index.
  1. Gastrointestinal system—Diseases—Handbooks, manuals, etc. I. Title. [DNLM: 1.
Gastrointestinal Diseases. WI 100 H168k]
RC801.H27   1986   616.3'3   86-22670
ISBN-13: 978-0-306-42309-3   e-ISBN-13: 978-1-4684-1251-2
DOI: 10.1007/978-1-4684-1251-2

Dedicated to my parents, Chaya and Shalom Halevy;
my wife, Adina; and my children, Ilit, Itai, Noam, and Dan,
who each in their own way made the writing
of this book possible.

.

Foreword

This book is an extraordinary achievement by Jonathan Halevy. To condense the material of three major gastrointestinal textbooks would be triumph enough, but to add a distillate of the contents of ten journals, from 1980 to 1985, requires Herculean vigor. To reorganize all the material under headings which extract concise "facts" from wheat and chaff requires a passionate interest in patients together with an understanding of physiology. Fortunately, Jonathan Halevy has just the right combination of clinical and laboratory interest for him to select the details of what is important. Such compulsive dedication has now made it possible for the practicing physician, gastroenterologist, or house officer, interested in preparing for board examinations or simply browsing in the field, to have at his fingertips a series of definitions and to put in his pocket the key facts for diagnosis and therapy.

Of course, facts by themselves are something of which to be a little wary. Scientists first, doctors regard facts the way farmers look at sheep—to be sheared for their utility. Medicine too often is only a fact-gathering occupation (some lectures send me to woolgathering), in which having the facts sometimes clouds clinical judgment about what is important for the individual patient. Rationalism and romanticism lie at the two poles of medical practice, but rationalism rules in the 1980s. If you define intuition, as I do, as the immediate apprehension of an idea or concept, to rely on intuition you have to have a great many conscious and even preconscious facts at your disposal. Indeed, some would argue that intuition is nothing more than the very rapid search for facts on a preconscious level to come up with a feeling or judgment. That is what clinicians do much of the time. If that is so, then Dr. Halevy has given us a foundation not only for judgment but also for intuition. If the average GI fellow at Yale had at his command the incredible array of data present in this book, he could teach his teachers. And he would be a better doctor for it.

The year 1985 marked the 75th anniversary of the Flexner report. Flexner recognized that there were two kinds of facts: those apprehended by chemistry, physics, and biology (the kinds of facts that we teach in medical school), and another kind of fact, dealt with by "different apperceptive and appreciative apparatus." The latter had to do with cultural experience, something that Flexner took for granted, but which his followers have ignored in favor of logically observed data and the reports of what William James called the "brass band industry." By that James meant the instruments which we use for measuring and recording objective, as opposed to subjective, reports. Still, facts are as useful to the physician as any instrument. Indeed, the uncovering of those facts over the past 100 years has been responsible for the major advances against disease. After he absorbs the information in this book, I hope that the reader will have the leisure to remember that medicine is both science and art. Physicians treat persons in whom personal, social, and psychological components influence how the perturbations of the cell that we call disease are reflected in illness. Medicine needs both models, the reductionist medical–materialist model and the intuitive–romantic one. In this book we learn the facts so that we can become better clinicians by spending more time with our patients.

This book will prove of value to the medical student learning gastroenterology, to the resident who wants a *vade mecum* within reach in his forays with the gastroenterologists, and to every GI fellow. I am grateful to Plenum for putting the book out so rapidly, so cheaply, and so wisely. I congratulate Jonathan on his achievement.

Howard M. Spiro, M.D.

New Haven, Connecticut

Preface

As in all other fields of medicine, basic knowledge and newer developments in gastroenterology are made available, to those interested, in the form of detailed and well-written textbooks that present a comprehensive approach to this field.

This work is a concise compilation of facts that have important clinical relevance. It is designed to serve residents, internists, and gastroenterologists in practice when they are in need of an "immediate answer" to a practical problem arising in their day-to-day practice, and also for physicians preparing for the Board examinations in internal medicine or gastroenterology. The *key facts* in this book are based on information derived from the major textbooks in gastroenterology and liver disease, namely *Gastrointestinal Disease (Third Edition)*, edited by Sleisenger and Fordtran, Spiro's *Clinical Gastroenterology (Third Edition)*, and Sherlock's *Diseases of the Liver and Biliary System (Sixth Edition)*, and from the following journals: *Gastroenterology, Hepatology, Gut, Digestive Diseases and Sciences, American Journal of Gastroenterology, Scandinavian Journal of Gastroenterology, Journal of Clinical Gastroenterology, Diseases of the Colon and Rectum, Lancet,* and *Annals of Internal Medicine.*

For the sake of simplicity, I have not used subheadings in the book, but each *key fact* usually covers one aspect of a physiopathological or clinical entity. Important diseases or syndromes are covered by a few key facts. The central theme of each key fact has been *italicized* and, in looking for specific information, the reader should consult the Index. Key facts on related topics are grouped together for easy and logical review. I decided not to use references for each key fact because, to a large extent, the key facts contain information based on a few sources (textbooks and/or recent papers), and referring to all sources would have made the text lengthy and complicated. For further elucidation on each key fact, the reader should refer to the indexes of the above-named textbooks and/or to *Index Medicus* 1980–1985 using one of the key words in the specific key fact.

   I wish to thank my esteemed teacher, Howard M. Spiro, for his continued support.

Jonathan Halevy, M.D.

Tel Aviv, Israel

Contents

Key Facts in Gastroenterology

1
The Esophagus

1. In the relaxed state, the pressure in midesophagus is 5–10 mm Hg below ambient pressure—same as intrathoracic pressure.

2. The *venous drainage of the esophagus* is in the (a) upper third to the superior vena cava; (b) middle third to the azygos; and (c) lower third to portal vein via short gastric veins.

3. The most common *tracheoesophageal fistula* is the upper end of the esophagus, which ends in a blind sac and the lower end inserts posteriorly into the trachea (85–90%). The least common is an H–type fistula.

4. *Upper esophageal sphincter (UES)* is located at the level of C6, has a high resting pressure of 33 mm Hg, and is 3–5 cm long.

5. *Elevation of lower esophageal sphincter (LES) pressure* is caused by gastrin (probably not important physiologically), bombesin, motilin, pitressin, and metoclopramide. *Relaxation of LES* is caused by secretin, CCK, glucagon, progesterone, peppermint, alcohol, smoking, and theophylline. No effect on LES pressure has been demonstrated by somatostatin and VIP.

6. *LES relaxation* after deglutition is at least partially controlled by the vagus. However, vagotomy does *not* affect LES pressure.

7. *Primary peristalsis*: a swallow initiates a monophasic wave that begins below the cricopharyngeus and sweeps down to the LES zone. *Secondary peristalsis*: aperistaltic contraction stimulated by distention (material remaining in the esophagus or that has been refluxed into it).

8. Prolonged *spasm of UES* may lead to inflammatory polyps of vocal cords and trachea.

9. The following are suggestive of *dysphagia of motor origin*: (a) intermittency; (b) production by either solids or liquids (mainly cold liquids); (c) relief by repeated swallowing or the Valsalva maneuver; and (d) intensification by stress.

10. *Wet swallow* (10 ml) is followed by a peristaltic wave of higher amplitude compared with the wave that follows a dry swallow.

11. *Dysphagia* is common after radical neck dissection for carcinoma of the larynx.

12. *Myotomy of UES* may relieve severe neuromuscular dysphagia, but if stenosis occurs as a complication of surgery it is very difficult to treat surgically.

13. In *achalasia*, dysphagia is produced by both solids and liquids and is made worse by stress or rapid eating, nocturnal regurgitation is common, and odynophagia is occasionally seen.

14. In *achalasia*, disappearance of gastric bubble is common, and concomitant *epiphrenic diverticle* may be observed occasionally.

15. Manometric findings in *achalasia*: (a) elevated resting pressure; (b) deglutition causes broad low-amplitude simultaneous pressure waves with no peristalsis; and (c) high resting pressure in LES with a significant sphincter–stomach gradient remaining after deglutition.

16. *Squamous cell carcinoma* is diagnosed in 2–7% of cases of *achalasia*—more if untreated.

17. A difficult differential diagnosis: *achalasia* and infiltrating *carcinoma of gastroesophageal (GE) junction*; endoscopy with biopsy is indicated.

18. Clinical trials of *calcium channel blockers* (verapamil, nifedipine) or nitrites in achalasia show equivocal results at this writing.

19. *Treatment of achalasia*: pneumatic dilatation or surgical myotomy. Myotomy probably carries higher success rates but also higher rates of gastroesophageal reflux as a complication.

20. When a perforation is suspected after *pneumatic dilatation* in achalasia, it should be excluded by water-soluble contrast material.

21. *Contraindications to balloon dilatation in achalasia* are (a) a noncooperative patient; (b) recent myocardial infarction; and (c) inability to exclude carcinoma. Relative contraindications include (a) tortuous esophagus; (b) previous myotomy; (c) previous unsuccessful dilatation; and (d) infancy.

22. In *diffuse esophageal spasm (DES)*: (a) there is a diffuse muscular thickening of the lower two-thirds of the esophagus, (b) dysphagia and pain are triggered by cold or warm food, (c) manometry reveals an increase in baseline pressure with high-amplitude spontaneous *simultaneous* contractions, and (d) "nutcracker esophagus" is a manometric (and radiologic) variant with very high-amplitude contractions in lower esophagus.

23. A point to *differentiate DES from achalasia*: LES has normal contraction and relaxation in DES.

24. *Treatment of DES* is disappointing: (a) nitrites or nifedipine; (b) pneumatic dilatation (45% relief compared with 80% relief in achalasia); and (c) long myotomy as a last-resort procedure.

25. In *scleroderma*: (a) there is absence of esophageal peristalsis with weak or no response to wet swallow; (b) slow esophageal and gastric emptying are demonstrated in scintigraphic studies; (c) LES is hypotonic; (d) dysphagia is common; (e) reflux symptoms may occur; (f) wide-mouthed diverticula in esophagus and colon are typical; and (g) there is no association with esophageal carcinoma.

26. In *diabetic neuropathy*, the esophagus demonstrates clinical and manometric features similar to those in scleroderma.

27. *Manometry is diagnostic* in (a) achalasia; (b) DES; (c) scleroderma; and (d) incompetent LES.

28. *Regurgitation* is defined as reflux that has passed UES that the patient has become aware of (stains a pillow, fluid in mouth, or aspiration).

29. *LES pressure* is not in good correlation with reflux, but chances of reflux are increased when it is below 7 mm Hg.

30. *Inappropriate relaxation of LES* is probably the most important factor in the pathophysiology of reflux.

31. *Agents that promote reflux*: estrogen, progesterone, diazepam (Valium), morphine (Demerol), and theophylline.

32. *Heartburn* is the most common symptom of reflux, *dysphagia* is more common than *odynophagia*, and bleeding is uncommon.

33. *Reflux symptoms* are common at night because of decreased frequency of swallowing—less peristalsis is induced to remove the refluxed fluids.

34. The presence of *hiatus hernia* is not a prerequisite for reflux, and its presence or absence has no implications for the medical management of reflux.

35. The *PH probe* (in lower esophagus) is the most sensitive diagnostic test for the existence of reflux.

36. *Bernstein test* is sensitive in assessing the relationship between reflux and the patient's symptoms.

37. *Esophageal histology in reflux*: (a) thickened basal layer (>15% of mucosal thickness); and (b) dermal pegs extend almost to the surface.

38. *Complications of reflux*: (a) stricture; (b) Barret's esophagus; and (c) esophageal ulcer (uncommon).

39. *Stricture* causes progressive dysphagia—uncomplicated reflux esophagitis causes nonprogressive dysphagia.

40. Three types of columnar epithelium are possible in *Barret's esophagus*: (a) *columnar* (intestinal type with villi and goblet cells—the most common); (b) *fundal gastric type* (with parietal and chief cells); and (c) *junctional type* (with cardiac mucous cells).

41. In *Barret's esophagus*, there is a 10% chance of the development of adenocarcinoma. Annual endoscopy with cytology is recommended. In contrast to this "traditional" prevalence, a recent study reports the occurrence of two cases of adenocarcinoma during a mean follow-up of 20 years in 105 patients with Barret's esophagus (Spechler SJ et al, Gastroenterology 87:927, 1984).

42. *Barret's esophagus* has been reported in children with reflux esophagitis (Dahms BB & Rothstein FC, Gastroenterology 86:318, 1984).

43. *Ulcers in Barret's esophagus* respond to H_2-blockers but not to antacids.

44. *Esophageal ulceration* is characterized by intense continuous pain; it may lead to severe hematemesis, but perforation is uncommon.

45. *Medical management of gastroesophageal reflux* includes (a) elevation of the head of the bed (on 6- to 8-inch blocks); (b) avoidance of citrus juice, alcohol, smoking, and excess fat in diet; (c) weight reduction; and (d) betanechol, metoclopramide, antacids (Gaviscon is probably preferred), and H_2-blockers.

46. *Surgery should be considered in gastroesophageal reflux* when one of the following is diagnosed: (a) stricture; (b) significant bleeding; (c) aspiration; or (d) intractability.

47. Ninety percent of patients with *benign esophageal stricture* will benefit from dilatation combined with antireflux therapy.

48. *Complications of surgery for gastroesophageal reflux* are (a) recurrence; (b) obstruction at the site of repair; (c) gastric ulcers; and (d) fistula.

49. If *fundoplication* is impossible or when the extent of esophageal damage is extensive, interposition of colon or jejunum should be considered; however, it is associated with a 10–15% mortality.

50. When significant *symptoms of reflux with Barret's esophagus* are present, antireflux surgery should be considered, but regression postsurgery was demonstrated in only 40% of cases. Fundoplication prevents new esophageal strictures and improves symptoms from existing strictures.

51. *Paraesophageal hernia* does not lead to reflux, but it does cause bleeding and occasional *gastric volvulus*.

52. *Alcohol* has a direct cause-and-effect relationship to esophagitis. Hard liquor produces more symptoms than does beer.

53. *Nonsteroidal antiinflammatory drugs (NSAID)* are associated with benign esophageal stricture (Wilkins WE et al, Gut 25:478, 1984).

54. *Plummer–Vinson syndrome,* or *Paterson–Brown–Kelly syndrome,* is characterized by webs in the upper 2–4 cm of the esophagus with iron deficiency anemia. *Dysphagia* and pulmonary symptoms are common. *Hypopharyngeal or esophageal carcinoma* will develop in 50% of cases.

55. *Lower esophageal ring,* or *Schatzki's ring,* is a thin luminal narrowing in distal esophagus that leads to intermittent dysphagia but that can also be asymptomatic.

56. *Stricture induced by nasogastric (N-G) tube* is uncommon in the absence of preexisting esophagitis.

57. *Leiomyomas of the esophagus* are mostly discovered as incidental findings in upper GI series or endoscopy. They rarely bleed and may be multiple.

58. *Squamous cell carcinoma of the esophagus* (esophageal Ca) has a high incidence in North China and the Caspian region. In the United States, it is more common in urban areas than in rural regions.

59. *Squamous cell Ca* is associated with (a) chronic irritation (stricture, achalasia, irradiation, reflux); (b) alcohol; (c) smoking; (d) tylosis; and (e) celiac sprue.

60. Aperistalsis with abnormal manometric findings in LES may be present in *esophageal carcinoma*.

61. *Esophageal Ca* has a tendency toward contiguous spread due to lack of a serosal layer in the esophagus.

62. *Complications of esophageal carcinoma* include (a) aspiration pneumonitis (most common); (b) tracheoesophageal fistula; (c) esophageobronchial or esophageopleural fistulas; and (d) erosion of the tumor into the aorta with exanguination (extremely rare).

63. *Staging of esophageal carcinoma* is best accomplished with a computed tomographic (CT) scan, which can demonstrate even slight mucosal thickening.

64. Before *surgical management of esophageal carcinoma*, one should perform (a) sonography of liver to exclude metastases; (b) examination of vocal cords; and (c) bronchoscopy.

65. *Hypercalcemia* is common in squamous cell tumor of the esophagus—ectopic parathyroid hormone (PTH)?

66. The preferred *management of esophageal squamous cell carcinoma* is controversial—in 600 patients, there was no advantage to surgery over irradiation or over combination therapy.

67. *A common practical approach toward esophageal carcinoma* is irradiation for upper esophageal tumors and surgery for lower tumors or adenocarcinoma of the cardiac region. A prosthesis is used for palliation when it becomes difficult to maintain a patent lumen.

68. *Bouginage* is the preferred *approach to benign esophageal stricture* developing after irradiation from squamous cell carcinoma.

69. *Five-year survival for esophageal carcinoma* is about 9% following any mode of therapy. Prognosis is poorest in upper esophageal tumor. Prognosis is better in Japan (5-year survival of 18.4%).

70. *Melanoma* may present as an esophageal polyp.

71. *Zenker* and *epiphrenic diverticles* are pulsion diverticles—probably the result of motility disturbance.

72. *Midesophageal diverticle* is a traction diverticle—probably the result of both motility disturbances and fibrous adhesions following infective processes (such as mediastinal node tuberculosis).

73. *Esophageal pseudodiverticles* are small and multiple. They are associated with upper stricture (which should be dilated) and with candida infections.

74. In *esophageal candidiasis*, whether localized or as part of chronic mucocutaneous candidiasis, dysphagia is more prominent than odynophagia and strictures may develop.

75. *Esophageal candidiasis* should be verified by silver methenamine stain of mycelia in material obtained by exfoliative cytology.

76. *Herpetic esophagitis* (a) is common in lymphoma and leukemia; (b) may be present in healthy persons; and (c) may demonstrate esophageal ulcers on esophagram.

77. In *graft-versus-host disease*, esophageal involvement is common, with odynophagia, dysphagia, stricture, and webs.

78. *Mallory–Weiss syndrome* is (a) found in 14% of patients hospitalized for upper GI bleeding; and (b) is most common on the right side of the lower esophageal wall.

79. *Boerhaave perforation* (a) is a tear through all the layers of the esophagus produced by a sudden increase in esophageal pressure; (b) occurs mostly in males after having a heavy meal; (c) is more common on the left lateral wall; and (d) can lead to left pleural effusion and subcutaneous emphysema in the neck.

80. *Serum amylase* is elevated in esophageal perforation.

81. Causes of *esophageal perforation* other than a heavy meal include (a) trauma (mainly motor vehicle accident); (b) gunshot wound; and (c) vigorous suctioning or attempts to feed by nasogastric tube in the newborn.

82. The use of *barium* is not contraindicated in esophageal perforations or lacerations, but granulomas will form.

83. Medical management of instrumental perforation of esophagus includes NPO, continuous suctioning, and antimicrobial agents. This approach has been found to be highly efficient when started early in the course.

84. *Foreign bodies in the esophagus* commonly pass easily to the stomach, except for coins, which tend to stop at the level of T1.

85. Tetracycline, KCl, edrophonium, and Clinitest tablets have all been shown to cause esophageal strictures.

2
The Stomach and Duodenum

1. *The stomach* has a volume of 150 ml (adult); the cardia is located 1 inch (2.5 cm) left of the midline at the level of T9. The greater curvature is 4–6 times longer than the smaller curvature and is more mobile; the pyloric channel is 1 inch long; the pylorus is 1 inch to the right of the midline at the level of L1.

2. *Blood supply to the stomach*: (a) *left gastric artery*, a branch of the celiac artery, supplies the lower third of the esophagus, the upper part of the stomach, and the lesser curvature; (b) *right gastric artery*, a branch of hepatic artery, supplies the lower part of the stomach; (c) *short gastric arteries*, from the splenic artery in the hilus of the spleen, supply the fundus; and (d) *left gastroepiploic artery*, from the gastroduodenal branch of the hepatic artery, supplies the lower part of the greater curvature.

3. *The parasympathetic innervation* of the stomach is through the anterior and posterior nerves of Latarjet, branches of the vagus.

4. *Foveolae gastricae* are numerous pits (about 3.5 million) punctuating the innermost lining of the stomach.

4

5. *Cells in gastric glands*: (a) *chief* (zymogen); (b) *parietal* (oxyntic); (c) *mucous neck*; and (d) *endocrinelike*.

6. *Acid* and *intrinsic factor (IF)* are secreted by parietal cells.

7. *G cells* in the antrum secrete gastrin, ACTH-like peptide, and enkephalin–endorphine-related peptides.

8. *D cells* in stomach and pylorus secrete somatostatin.

9. *Relaxation of the smooth muscle of the stomach* is induced by neurotensin, VIP, norepinephrine, and high concentration of secretin.

10. The *proximal stomach* contracts only after stimulation. The *distal stomach* undergoes spontaneous peristalsis.

11. The *pacemaker region* of the stomach is high on the greater curvature (below the fundus). The pacemaker region has the fastest frequency of spontaneous depolarization (3/min in humans).

12. *Functions of the stomach* include (a) storage; (b) mixing and grinding; and (c) timely emptying.

13. *Gastric processing* results in food particles no larger than 1 mm reaching the duodenum.

14. *Liquids* have an emptying rate proportional to the volume remaining in the stomach, after a brief period of rapid emptying.

15. *Solids* empty from the stomach at a relatively constant rate that can be altered by the character of other ingested substances, such as fat or hypertonic fluids.

16. *Sugar* passes from the stomach to the duodenum at a constant rate of 2.13 kcal/min.

17. *Gastric emptying is reduced* by fat, acidity (in upper small intestine), and hyperosmotic contents.

18. *Vagotomy* slows gastric emptying of solids and accelerates emptying of fluids.

19. Clinically significant *delayed gastric emptying* has been demonstrated in *reflux esophagitis* and *viral gastroenteritis*. Metoclopramide decreases symptoms.

20. *Delayed gastric emptying* of a solid meal or barium is common in *diabetic neuropathy*. Metoclopramide is helpful.

21. *Psychogenic vomiting* occurs after starting the meal or immediately upon its completion.

22. *Sodium bicarbonate* is useful to relieve nausea. Up to 1/2 teaspoon is safe. Much larger amounts may cause gastric rupture by the gas formed in the stomach.

23. *Basal acid output (BAO)* is defined as the amount of acid secreted per hour under basal conditions (measured by gastric aspiration). *Maximal acid output (MAO)* is defined as the sum of four 15-min acid outputs following the administration of pentagastrin or histamine. *Peak acid output (PAO)* is defined as the sum of the two highest consecutive 15-min acid outputs following the administration of pentagastrin or histamine multiplied by two. MAO reflects parietal cell mass; it may decrease by 50–60% after vagotomy.

24. *BAO* in males: 0–17 mmol/hr; in females: 0–7.1 mmol/hr; BAO/PAO averages 0.07–0.08 in both males and females.

25. BAO is minimal between 5 and 11 a.m., maximal between 2 and 11 p.m.

26. *Phases of food-stimulated acid secretion* include (a) cephalic-vagal (thought, smell, sight, taste); (b) distention; and (c) chemical reaction of food with gastric mucosa. The vagus is important in (a) and (b).

27. *Proteins* and their hydrolytic products are potent stimulants of acid secretion when eaten or given intravenously (release gastrin). *Carbohydrates* and *fat* decrease acid output (mechanism unknown).

28. *Secretin* and *glucagon* inhibit gastric secretion.

29. *Opiates* and *calcium* stimulate gastric secretion.

30. *Secretin, gastrin, CCK,* and *enterogastrone* decrease gastric emptying.

31. All the following beverages increase gastric acid output compared with water: Sanka, Coca-Cola, 7-Up, tea, coffee, Tab, beer, and milk.

32. When antral pH decreases below 2.5–3.0, antral gastrin release is suppressed.

33. *Serum pepsinogen I* reflects MAO because it is secreted only by oxyntic glandular mucosa.

34. The mucus covering gastric mucosa (a) is 95% water, 5% glycoprotein; (b) serves as a lubricant; and (c) probably slows inward H diffusion.

35. HCO_3 is secreted by oxyntic mucosa in the stomach, as well as in the pyloric region and duodenum. NSAID, alcohol, and bile salts reduce HCO_3 secretions by the stomach.

36. Histological classification of *nonerosive gastritis*: (a) *superficial gastritis*: inflammatory cells in foveolar region; (b) *atrophic gastritis*: inflammatory cells invade glandular area with mild to moderate destruction of glands; and (c) *gastric atrophy*: no inflammatory cells, destruction of all or most of the glands.

37. *Intestinal metaplasia* is common in severe forms of nonerosive gastritis.

38. *Nonerosive gastritis* is a histological entity with no clinical implications except for occasional epigastric pain aggravated by food and relieved by antacid.

39. The mucosa usually appears normal on endoscopy in *nonerosive gastritis*.

40. *Superficial gastritis* is present in 33% of the population at age 30. The prevalence increases with age, as does the histological progress to atrophic gastritis.

41. *Nonerosive gastritis* is universal following partial gastrectomy.

42. *Type A atrophic gastritis* is found only in the fundus; antiparietal cell antibodies are present, associated with pernicious anemia, autoimmune thyroid disease, and diabetes; also, gastrin levels are high. This type of gastritis occurs in 20% of whites. *Type B atrophic gastritis* is a diffuse process considered to reflect a wear-and-tear phenomenon associated with low gastrin levels. Ten percent of those affected have antibodies against gastrin-producing cells. This type of gastritis occurs in 5% of the general population.

43. *Atrophic gastritis* is a forerunner of gastric cancer in 10% of patients carefully followed.

44. *Vitiligo* is common in atrophic gastritis.

45. *Hypertrophic gastritis* includes (a) glandular type (with hyperchlorhydria); (b) Menetrier's (with achlorhydria in 75%); and (c) Zollinger–Ellison syndrome.

46. In *Menetrier's disease*, or *giant hypertrophic gastritis*, (a) the antrum is spared; (b) patients may have nonspecific ulcerlike symptoms; (c) there is loss of albumin, globulin, transferrin, and folic acid; (d) the onset may be part of the multiple endocrine neoplasia (MEN) syndrome; (e) there is probably a 10% risk of gastric carcinoma; and (f) the thickened gastric folds can be demonstrated by ultrasound or CT scan.

47. In *pernicious anemia*, (a) gastrin is elevated in 80% of cases; (b) antiparietal cell antibodies are present in 90% of cases (20% prevalence in healthy patients over age 60); (c) anti-IF antibodies are present in 60%; (d) antithyroid antibodies are present in 50%; (e) severe fundic gland atrophy with pseudopyloric and intestinal metaplasia is common; (f) there is a familial tendency; and (g) there is an increased incidence of gastric carcinoma.

48. Types of *eosinophilic gastroenteritis*: (a) *mucosal*: associated with anemia, malabsorption, and protein loss; (b) *muscular*: associated with pyloric and small bowel obstruction; and (c) *subserosal*: characterized by "eosinophilic" ascites. Background factors: food allergy, elevated IgE, eosinophilia (up to 80%). Treatment: steroids.

49. Streptococci are the commonest cause (50%) of *phlegmonous gastritis*.

50. In *gastric TB*, the diagnosis is made by the finding of acid-fast bacilli or caseating granulomas in the stomach. Cultures from gastric secretions are commonly negative.

51. A dramatic unexplained decrease in the *incidence of gastric cancer* in the United States has occurred during the past four decades.

52. *Achlorhydria* predisposes to a high concentration of nitrite-forming bacteria in the stomach (gastric carcinogens).

53. High salt consumption is associated with increased incidence of *gastric carcinoma*.

54. *Gastric carcinoma* is more common in patients with blood group A and in relatives of patients with this carcinoma (× 2–3).

55. *Incidence of gastric carcinoma* is increased in acquired hypogammaglobulinemia and in celiac disease (where there is IgA deficiency).

56. The presence of *duodenal ulcer* decreases the *risk of gastric carcinoma* about tenfold.

57. The overall incidence of gastric carcinoma after Billroth surgery (I or II) is 3%. The incidence increases with time after surgery. Endoscopy every 3–5 years starting from 15 years after surgery is recommended.

58. In one study, 31–39 years after subtotal gastrectomy for peptic ulcer disease (PUD), the prevalence of carcinoma in the remnant stomach was found to be threefold the expected prevalence. Patients operated on for gastric ulcer were more susceptible to this complication (Pickford IR et al, Gut 25:393, 1984).

59. *Gastric carcinoma* always originates from mucus cells, never from parietal or chief cells.

60. *Symptoms in gastric carcinoma:* (a) pain is the most common symptom; (b) hemorrhage or perforation are uncommon; (c) nausea and vomiting are common in advanced stage; (d) *protein loss* is possible; (e) *meningeal metastases* are characteristic; (f) *acanthosis nigricans* is very rare; and (g) *gastrocolic fistula* may occur.

61. In *gastric carcinoma*, 65% of patients have basal achlorhydria, but only 20–25% will have achlorhydria after stimulation of gastric acid secretion (e.g., by pentagastrin).

62. *Differential diagnosis of big gastric folds* includes (a) Menetrier; (b) lymphoma; (c) gastritis; and (d) carcinoma.

63. *Differential diagnosis of linitis plastica* includes (a) carcinoma; (b) Crohn's disease of the stomach; and (c) syphilis.

64. *Management of gastric carcinoma:* (a) resection of the tumor: if found to be resectable; (b) palliative surgery: in diffuse process when obstruction or hemorrhage occurs, otherwise chemotherapy; (c) resection of spleen and omentum as part of curative surgery; and (d) adjuvant chemotherapy: administered after curative resection (except in early gastric cancer, when it is unnecessary).

65. *Prognosis of gastric carcinoma*: (a) overall 5-year survival: 5–15%; one-year survival: 30–33%; after curative surgery, 5-year survival of 50% was observed; (b) 25–50% of patients are potential candidates for curative surgery; (c) prognosis is worse when the tumor is in the fundus; and (d) prognosis is worse for the young and elderly and is better for middle-age patients.

66. *Upper endoscopy* once a year is recommended after resection of gastric tumor because recurrence in the suture line is common.

67. *Gastric cytology* positive for malignancy is an indication for total gastrectomy even when a localized lesion cannot be detected.

68. *Metastases to the wall of the stomach* occur in 25% of melanomata and have been reported in breast and pancreatic tumors.

69. *Gastric lymphoma* is in itself rare but is the commonest among the extranodal lymphomas. It is mostly B-cell lymphoma of the diffuse histocytic variant.

70. *Five-year survival in gastric lymphoma*: 50%.

71. *Lymphoma* that spreads to the GI tract involves most frequently the pancreas and the stomach.

72. *Leiomyomas* are located mainly in the proximal stomach; they are usually asymptomatic. *Leiomyosarcoma* is located in all segments; 5-year survival of the latter is 25–30%.

73. *Gastric polyps* (a) are less common than colonic polyps; (b) may be *hyperplastic* (most common), *adenomatous* (more common in antrum), or *hamartomatous*; (c) rarely have symptoms (hemorrhage or pyloric obstruction); (d) are associated with achlorhydria (90%), atrophic gastritis, pernicious anemia, or gastric carcinoma (the latter is present in 33% of patients with multiple polyps); (e) are more common after Billroth surgery; and (f) may be part of the colon polyposis syndrome.

74. *Solitary gastric polyps* occur most commonly in the pyloric canal and next most commonly along the lesser curvature.

75. In *pernicious anemia*, gastric polyps are more common than carcinoma.

76. *Indications for surgery in gastric polyposis* include (a) an adenomatous polyp larger than 2 cm that cannot be removed endoscopically; (b) a sessile polyp with equivocal endoscopic diagnosis (some authorities include any sessile polyp); and (c) any symptomatic polyp.

77. Triad of *acute gastric volvulus*: (a) violent retching but no vomitus, (b) constant, severe epigastric pain; and (c) difficulty in advancing nasogastric tube.

78. Predisposing factors for *gastric bezoars* include incomplete mastication, hypochlorhydria, reduced antral motility, and previous Billroth surgery (I or II, especially with vagotomy), possibly cimetidine.

79. *Infantile hypertrophic pyloric stenosis* occurs in 1 of 250 births; M/F: 3–4/1.

80. *Congenital duodenal atresia* or *stenosis* occurs mostly distal to the ampulla of Vater (in 80% of cases).

81. The most common reason for *duodenal obstruction* in childhood is *intestinal malrotation*.

82. *Double bubble sign* in plain abdominal film is indicative of duodenal obstruction.

83. In *annular pancreas* stenosing the duodenum, the preferred surgical approach is bypass surgery.

84. Types of *stress ulcers*: (a) *Cushing*, in intracranial disease; ulcers are deep, may perforate, and are associated with hyperchlorhydria; (b) *Curling*, in severe burns; ulcers are shallow and tend to bleed;

and (c) *drug-induced*, similar to Curling, but massive bleeding is less common.

85. *Steroid therapy and ulcers*: in 14% of patients taking more than 10 mg prednisone for 6 months, gastric ulcer will develop, mainly on lesser curvature, with little pain. It may present as bleeding or perforation. Total prednisone dose of more than 1 g is also associated with increased risk.

86. *Steroid-induced ulcers* are more common in rheumatoid arthritis than in other disorders treated with steroids.

87. Endoscopic evidence of mucosal injury was found in 50% of patients on *aspirin*.

88. Eighty percent of *stress ulcers* will stop bleeding following *gastric lavage* with cold saline. Vasoconstrictors in the lavage fluid offer no advantage.

89. In patients susceptible to the development of *stress ulcers*, prophylactic H_2-blockers or antacids are recommended.

90. A recent study reported a decrease in M/F ratio for *PUD* from 2:1 in 1968 to 1.3:1 today in admission rates and mortality (Kurata JH et al, Gastroenterology 88:96, 1985).

91. Ten percent of American males and 4% of females will suffer from *duodenal ulcer (DU)* during their lifetime.

92. In 73% of *DU* patients, scanning electron microscopy demonstrated bacillus bacteria attached to mucosal gastric cells.

93. *Aspirin* is a major causative factor in *gastric ulcer (GU)* but not in DU.

94. *Acetaminophen* given orally protects gastric mucosa from damage by aspirin or alcohol, probably by increasing *prostacycline*.

95. *Smoking* definitely delays healing of DU and may increase prevalence.

96. Compared with the general population, *DU* is 30% more common in blood group O and 50% more common in nonsecretors of blood antigens in saliva.

97. *Pepsinogen I* is elevated in 30–50% of cases of *DU*.

98. The mode of inheritance of *DU* is not clear, but DU has been found in 16 of 85 relatives of DU patients.

99. *Familial DU* had been described in families with *rapid gastric emptying,* with *childhood or early-onset DU,* and with *combined DU and GU.*

100. *Gastric acid secretion* is necessary for the development of DU. DU is uncommon when MAO is less than 10 mmol/hr.

101. *Fasting serum gastrin* is normal in most patients with DU.

102. Only one-third of patients with *DU* have elevated MAO. There is much overlap with normals.

103. *Mechanisms for maintaining mucosal integrity:* (a) cell renewal; (b) mucus production; (c) HCO_3 secretion; (d) blood flow; and (e) prostaglandin production.

104. *Decreased incidence of duodenal ulcer* is found in (a) type A gastritis; (b) autoimmune polyglandular syndromes (e.g., Addison's disease, type I diabetes); and (c) hypertension.

105. *Qualities of DU pain:* (a) rhythmicity; (b) periodicity; and (c) chronicity.

106. Pain radiating to RUQ in DU suggests *pyloric channel* or *postbulbar ulcer.*

107. In *DU* there is no correlation between disappearance of symptoms and ulcer healing.

108. *Activity of a DU* is defined by symptoms and not by radiography.

109. *Dyspepsia* is characterized by fullness, discomfort, or a burning sensation in the epigastrium, often accompanied by belching and bloating. Most patients with dyspepsia do not have obvious pathology in the upper GI or biliary tract.

110. *Moynihan's syndrome*: patients with dyspepsia and pain characteristics as in DU but no ulcer crater can be demonstrated. Persistent symptoms should be treated as if a DU were present.

111. *Giant DU*: (a) larger than 2.5 cm; (b) mostly in posterior wall; (c) higher rate of penetration and hemorrhage; and (d) simulates deformed bulb or a diverticle on roentgenogram.

112. In *pyloric channel ulcers*, (a) pain is triggered by food; (b) there is no relief with antacids; and (c) vomiting is frequent.

113. *Postbulbar ulcers* (a) are easy to miss on radiographic or endoscopic examination; (b) bleed in two-thirds of cases; and (c) are commonly associated with intractability and obstruction.

114. The preferred *initial diagnostic approach in suspected DU* is controversial; most authorities agree that both double-contrast radiography and endoscopy are sensitive. The former is less costly but somewhat less sensitive.

115. Once the diagnosis of DU has been made, *endoscopy* is not indicated to evaluate the response to therapy or the recurrence of symptoms similar to the initial attack.

116. The study of *gastric secretory capacity* is obsolete in evaluating PUD, or any other disorder.

117. *Indications for evaluation of serum gastrin levels*: (a) in a child or an adolescent with DU; (b) when Z-E is suspected; (c) in any patient with a family history of duodenal ulcer combined with endocrine abnormalities.

118. "Once an ulcer always an ulcer" is not a true statement—within 15 years after presentation with DU (in Fry's series) two-thirds were symptom free, 14% bled, 8% had perforation, and 1 of 265 died of DU.

119. *Coffee, tea, milk,* and many other beverages are strong secretagogues. There is no need to avoid them completely in DU, but moderation of consumption, especially on an empty stomach, is recommended.

120. *Calcium* is a strong gastric secretagogue.

121. H_1 *receptors* are found in the skin, bronchi, nasal mucosa, and intestinal smooth muscle. H_2 *receptors* are found in gastric parietal cells, cardiac atrium, uterus, and T lymphocytes.

122. *Cimetidine*: Imidazole ring. *Ranitidine*: Furan ring.

123. *Side effects of cimetidine* include (a) painful gynecomastia (in 1%, dose dependent); (b) impotence (only in very high doses used in gastrinoma); (c) oligospermia; (d) psychiatric abnormalities; (e) bone marrow depression; (f) hypocalcemia (decreased PTH); (g) interstitial nephritis; (h) bradycardia and hypotension; and (i) reduced clearance of drugs (propranolol, diazepam, anticoagulants, lidocaine). These side effects are exceedingly rare. The experience with ranitidine is less extensive but it appears not to induce most of these side effects.

124. *Cimetidine* is excreted by the kidneys; the dose should be reduced in chronic renal failure.

125. *Cimetidine* seems to produce a prolonged suppression of pepsin, while fasting serum gastrin levels and pentagastrin-stimulated acid secretion return to normal 2 weeks after stopping H_2 blockers.

126. *Effects of antacids*: (a) neutralization of gastric acid; (b) reduced peptic activity, since pepsin is inactive in higher pH; and (c) binding of bile acids (the latter are considered ulcerogenic).

127. *Antacids* at bedtime are of short benefit because antacids leave an empty stomach very rapidly.

128. Preliminary studies indicate that *sucralfate* reduces the rate of recurrent ulcers compared with cimetidine and antacids (promotes scar formation?).

129. *Sucralfate* should be given 1 hr before meals, as it is neutralized by food.

130. *Omeprazole*, a gastric proton pump inhibitor, has a half-life in plasma of 50 min, but its effects last a few days after a single dose.

131. *Omeprazole* (30–60 mg/day) suppresses close to 100% of basal and stimulated acid secretion without an effect on pepsin secretion. It is currently used only on an experimental basis due to recent concern about induction of carcinoid tumors in animals.

132. In multiple studies, both *antacids* administered 1 and 3 hr after meals and at bedtime and *cimetidine* (1–1.2 g/day) produced healing of 78–96% of DU after 4 weeks of therapy compared with a 33–45% healing rate with placebo.

133. In *studies on H_2 blockers and sucralfate*: cimetidine 300 mg qid, 200 mg tid + 400 mg HS or 400 mg bid, and ranitidine 150 mg bid or sucralfate 1 g qid produced similar healing and recurrence rates.

134. Continuation of 400–800 mg *cimetidine* at bedtime or 400 mg bid over a 6- to 12-month period after healing of DU reduced ulcer recurrence rates to less than 20% (compared with 60–80% on placebo). Once H_2 blockers are stopped, the rate of recurrence is not reduced by a longer period of prior treatment.

135. *Ranitidine*, 150 mg bid, or a further course of *cimetidine*, 1 g/day, healed 63% of DU that were not healed on cimetidine, 1 g/day, administered for 6 weeks.

136. Fifty percent of *DU healed with cimetidine* will relapse within 1 year if maintenance therapy is not given.

137. For the patient on *maintenance therapy*, the duration of ulcer history and, to a lesser extent, the severity of symptoms of an individual attack correlate with relapse rate.

138. *Pirenzepine* is an anticholinergic drug with unique affinity to muscarinic receptors. Daily doses of 100–150 mg produce healing rates of DU similar to those with cimetidine (80–87%). A recent multicenter Austrian study showed that pirenzepine, 50 mg bid, and cimetidine, 1 g/day, were equally effective in healing DU (Procacciante F et al, Gut 25:178, 1984).

139. *Recommended management of symptomatic DU:* (a) initial treatment includes the choice between H_2 blockers, antacids, and sucralfate—the expected healing rate is 70–85% within 4–6 weeks; (b) if not healed within 6 weeks, treatment should be continued for 6 more weeks (50% will heal), or an alternative medication should be tried; and (c) in the event of recurrence, the therapeutic course should be repeated and continued with maintenance H_2 blockers (200–400 mg cimetidine or 150 mg ranitidine nightly).

140. Possible causes of *resistance to therapy in DU:* (a) poor compliance; (b) gastrinoma; (c) stress ulcer; and (d) smoking.

141. *Ranitidine,* a more potent inhibitor of acid secretion than cimetidine, has not yet proved more effective than cimetidine in the therapy of routine DU disease. It may offer an advantage over cimetidine in gastrinoma patients and possibly in other hypersecretory conditions that have failed to respond to cimetidine.

142. In the *initial treatment of DU,* there is no advantage in combining *H_2 blockers* with *antacids.* It may be advantagous in resistant ulcers and then they should not be taken at the same time, but doses should be separated by at least 1 hr.

143. Preliminary reports indicate that antacids plus cimetidine may reduce *rebleeding from duodenal ulcers.*

144. *Sucralfate* should not be added to H_2 blockers or to antacids, as it requires acid for dissolution in the stomach.

145. In any combination of *antiulcer therapy* (for DU), 20% of patients will not respond or will be very slow healers.

146. *Elective surgical management of DU* should be considered (a) when complications occur despite optimal medical care; (b) in failure to respond to optimal medical treatment; (c) in inability to continue medical therapy due to untoward side effects; and (d) in patients who have had two major complications of DU (i.e., two perforations, or perforation and a bleeding).

147. Patients who benefit most from *surgery for DU* are those with a long history of symptomatic DU with frequent recurrences and good remissions for a few months between recurrences and who are being operated on because of the onset of a major complication.

148. *Clinical DU* is three to four times more common than *gastric ulcer (GU)* but similar prevalence has been found in autopsies.

149. One-third of *GU* cases are related to *aspirin* (when more than 15 tablets a week are taken). *Alcohol* is also a predisposing factor.

150. On the average, *GU* occurs at an older age than does DU. It is more common in males.

151. *GU in the fundus* of the stomach is uncommon and is usually related to aspirin.

152. The lack of gastritis in the vicinity of GU points to an association with aspirin.

153. *Antral GU* tends to be smaller than GU in other regions of the stomach.

154. On the average, *gastric secretion* is decreased in GU, but most patients have normal gastric secretion. Similarly, serum gastrin levels are elevated, but its measurement is not indicated unless Z-E is suspected.

155. In *GU*, the more associated gastritis, the less gastric secretion.

156. A *GU close to the pylorus or associated with DU* is generally accompanied by hypersecretion.

157. Factors that may have a role in the *etiology of GU*: (a) back-diffusion of acid through breaks in the mucosa caused by aspirin, alcohol, or bile; (b) functional disturbance of the pylorus that fails to prevent bile reflux; and (c) delayed gastric emptying due to reduced antral motility.

147 ───

158. The current view is that *cancer* does not develop in a benign GU; if found, it was there to begin with.

159. When *GU is associated with DU*, the chances for malignancy in the GU are less.

160. In 30% of *GU*, the crater is infiltrated with *Candida*. It is harmless.

161. The *most common symptom of GU is abdominal pain*: (a) found usually in the epigastrium; (b) appears 1–3 hr after a meal; (c) sometimes aggravated by eating; (d) sometimes relieved by antacids; and (e) occurs at night in only 30% of cases.

162. *Weight loss is common in GU*, and nausea and vomiting are uncommon without obstruction.

163. *Bleeding in GU* is (a) common; (b) massive; and (c) more likely to recur than in DU.

164. It is controversial as to whether a *giant GU* (>2.0–2.5 cm) contains a malignant process more frequently than does a smaller GU or whether it simply heals more slowly.

165. Some workers perform endoscopy in every radiographically detected GU, as 3–7% of GU that appear to be benign on UGI series prove malignant. Others perform endoscopy only in GU that is atypical radiographically, larger than 2.5 cm, or resistant to therapy.

166. *Cytological studies* should never be forgotten in endoscopic evaluation of GU. It is recommended that at least seven biopsies be taken to exclude malignancy.

167. The healing process for GU is slower than for DU.

168. A recent multicenter study in Belgium indicated that *ranitidine* (300 mg/day) and *cimetidine* (1 g/day) brought about a similar *cure rate in GU*: 66% and 62% after 4 weeks of therapy and 78% and 87% after 6 weeks, respectively (The Belgium Peptic Ulcer Study Group, Gut 25:999, 1984).

169. In the *management of GU*: (a) "barrier breakers" (aspirin, NSAID, alcohol, smoking) are avoided; (b) H_2-blockers or antacids are given until the ulcer heals or for a maximun of 12–15 weeks; (c) endoscopy (or upper GI series) is performed after 8 weeks of therapy (some authorities recommend reendoscopy after 4–6 weeks); if healing is not complete, endoscopy should be repeated after 12 weeks; and (d) if GU does not heal after 15 weeks, surgery is indicated, even if no malignancy is found on biopsy.

170. *Endoscopy with biopsy* is indicated in *recurrence* of GU.

171. The current view is that *recurrences of GU*, even multiple ones, are not an indication for surgery.

172. *Indications for surgery in GU*: (a) carcinoma; (b) recurrence during treatment with H_2-blockers; (c) failure to heal after 12–15 weeks on medical therapy; and (d) recurrent bleeding or perforation.

173. *Maintenance dose of H_2-blockers* helps prevent recurrence in GU. However, recurrence will not develop in most patients, and maintenance is indicated initially only for Z-E, for elderly patients with systemic diseases in whom complications of GU develop, or in patients with rheumatoid arthritis on NSAID.

174. *Adverse effects of aspirin on the stomach*: (a) damage to the gastric mucosal barrier (the tight junction becomes permeable); and (b) inhibition of prostaglandin synthesis, depriving the stomach of their protective effects (i.e., increased mucus and HCO_3 production and increased mucosal blood flow).

175. Most of the *gastrin* in normal antrum and in gastrinoma tissue is G17, while most of the serum gastrin is G34.

176. In *Z-E*: (a) 60% of the tumors are malignant; (b) one-third are in the pancreas (more in the head and tail than in the body); (c) 13% are in the duodenal wall, with the rest in the splenic hilum, accessory pancreas, ovary, and parathyroid; (d) 50% of cases have multiple tumors; and (e) 25% are part of MEN I.

177. Seventy-five percent of *ulcers in Z-E* occur in the first part of the duodenum or in the stomach, some are found in the distal duodenum and in the jejunum.

178. Contrary to common opinion, most ulcers in Z-E are solitary. *Giant ulcers* do occur but are uncommon.

179. *Anastomotic ulcer* is very common in Z-E.

180. *One should suspect Z-E when there are:* (a) multiple ulcers; (b) ulcers distal to the first part of the duodenum; (c) refractory ulcers; (d) early recurrence after surgery; and (e) giant ulcers.

181. *Diarrhea is common in Z-E.* Possible causes: (a) acid is an osmotic laxative; (b) acid in the duodenum neutralizes lipase, leading to steatorrhea; (c) bile acids precipitate in acid pH; (d) gastrin inhibits fluid and electrolyte absorption; and (e) gastric metaplasia occurs in the jejunum and decreases absorptive surface.

182. Z-E manifesting as diarrhea with no ulcers occurs in 10% of Z-E patients.

183. *Z-E on upper GI series:* (a) thick folds in the stomach, the duodenum, and the small intestine; and (b) flocculation of barium due to its dilution by secretions.

184. *Normal fasting serum gastrin* level is 60–150 pg/ml. In Z-E >1000 pg/ml. However, in two-thirds of patients with pernicious anemia, levels above 1000 pg/ml were noted.

185. High *serum gastrin levels,* but usually <1000 pg/ml, can be found in atrophic gastritis, rheumatoid arthritis, vitiligo, diabetes mellitus, chronic renal failure, retained antrum, extensive intestinal resection, and pheochromocytoma.

186. When *Z-E* is suspected but serum gastrin is 150 pg/ml or less, stimulation tests should be conducted: (a) *intravenous secretin* increases serum gastrin only in Z-E (best test); (b) *intravenous calcium* increases serum gastrin levels in Z-E; and (c) standard meal will not increase serum gastrin or will increase its levels only modestly in Z-E.

187. Z-E (in contrast to pancreatic adenocarcinoma) is vascular, but celiac arteriography will demonstrate the tumor in only 20% of cases. CT scan is only somewhat better.

188. *Management of Z-E:* (a) high-dose H_2-blockers (1.5–2.5 times the regular dose) are given indefinitely; (b) surgery is not indicated because most tumors are multiple and difficult to detect; (c) in metastatic Z-E, streptozotocin (preferably intraarterial) and 5-fluorouracil (5-FU) are given; and (d) curative surgery is possible in 10% of cases, mainly in solitary extrapancreatic tumor.

189. The combination of *hyperparathyroidism* and *peptic ulcer disease (PUD)* suggests gastrinoma (Z-E).

190. The 10-year survival rate in Z-E is 30–40%.

191. *VIPOMA*, or *watery diarrhea and hypokalemia syndrome (WDHS)*, includes (a) non-beta islet cell tumor; (b) watery diarrhea with hypokalemia; and (c) no gastric hypersecretion (sometimes achlorhydria).

192. In 25% of *bleeding duodenal ulcers*, the bleeding is the presenting symptom of DU.

193. *Melena* is twice as common as *hematemesis* in DU. Melena and hematemesis have the same prevalence in GU.

194. Esophageal varices are the most common cuase of *persistent UGI bleeding*.

195. *Postural hypotension* is the most sensitive bedside tool for monitoring GI bleeding.

196. Fifty percent of patients with *Mallory–Weiss syndrome* have hiatus hernia.

197. In *DU* that has bled, the chance of recurrent bleeding is 30–50%, in *GU*, 6–40%. The rate of recurrent bleeding cannot be predicted either from the age of the patient or from the severity of the first bleeding episode.

198. After *surgery for bleeding ulcer,* 25% will rebleed from *anastomotic ulcer* or *gastritis.*

199. The following are commonly described *endoscopic stigmata* that may signify high risk of continued or recurrent bleeding in PUD: (a) visible vessel (50% recurrence); (b) oozing; (c) adherent blood clot; and (d) black spots on the crater.

200. *Predictors of a poor prognosis in bleeding PUD* include (a) old age; (b) other diseases (mainly liver); and (c) absence of drug or alcohol abuse history.

201. *Ulcer pain* frequently disappears when bleeding starts because acid is neutralized by blood.

202. *Hyperperistalsis* in upper GI bleeding is evidence for a significant bleeding.

203. Indications for *elective surgery* in *bleeding* PUD include (a) a second major bleed; (b) first major bleed plus history of intractability, obstruction, or perforation; (c) gastrinoma; and (d) planned kidney transplantation.

204. *Criteria for major bleeding in PUD:* (a) Hb < 10 g/dl and Hct < 28%; (b) clinical shock; and (c) more than 1500 ml whole blood required to restore blood volume.

205. The finding of *blood in the stomach* (on N-G tube: more than 10 ml gross blood, 30 ml dark guaiac-positive fluid, or 30 ml pink blood-flecked material) excludes the lower gut as the source of bleeding.

206. In 20–25% of patients, the *source of GI bleeding* is never discovered.

207. *Massive GI bleeding* still carries an 8–10% mortality but mainly in the aged or in those who have other severe illnesses.

208. In 85% of cases of *upper GI bleeding,* the cause is PUD (GU or gastritis, 50%; DU, 25%; reflux esophagitis, 25%).

209. *Arguments for performing urgent endoscopy in acute UGI bleeding:* (a) locates the site of bleeding in 80–85% of cases; (b) permits planning for early surgery or to delay surgery (the former in GU and the latter in bleeding erosive gastritis); (c) permits the selective use of angiography or vasopressin; (d) directs the surgeon if surgery is needed; and (e) helps in long-term planning—bleeding erosive gastritis will not be counted as a bleeding episode from an ulcer when considering surgery in a subsequent episode of upper GI bleeding.

210. A rise in *BUN* indicates considerable blood loss from upper GIT. BUN usually falls to normal within 12 hr after the bleeding has stopped.

211. The stool can stay black up to 10–12 days after cessation of the bleeding, and occult blood may be positive up to 2 weeks.

212. In *bleeding ulcers*, consideration of early surgery is suggested for: (a) gastric or postbulbar ulcers (tend to recur); (b) elderly patients; and (c) a patient who stopped bleeding and started again while in the hospital.

213. *Perforation* occurs in 10% of patients hospitalized for PUD; it is more frequent in males.

214. *The common site of perforation:* in DU, anterior wall of the first part of the duodenum; in GU, 60% are on the lesser curvature.

215. In one-third of patients with *perforation*, it is the first symptom of PUD.

216. *Mortality in perforation:* in GU 10–40%; in DU 5–13%; it is increased in: (a) the elderly; (b) females; (c) when surgery is delayed for more than 12 hr.

217. In *contained perforation* into the lesser sac, the iliac fossa, or into the anterior retroperitoneal plane, air may not be present under the diaphragm.

218. *Gastrografin* is preferred over barium to locate the site of perforation.

219. *Ulcer symptoms* frequently intensify before the onset of perforation.

220. *Penetration* is usually manifested by (a) back pain; (b) loss of the regular pattern of ulcer pain; (c) pain that becomes intractable to medical management; and (d) refractory night pain which recurs many times each night.

221. *Complete obstruction from PUD* is commonly preceded by symptoms of partial obstruction.

222. *Early signs of pyloric obstruction in PUD:* (a) ulcer pain early in the morning; and (b) pain refractory to antacids (because the stomach contains large amounts of acid).

223. In *pyloric obstruction,* serum gastrin levels may be as high as in Z-E.

224. *Management of pyloric obstruction in PUD:* (a) gastric decompression for at least 72 hr; (b) correction of fluid and electrolyte imbalance; (c) intravenous cimetidine; and (d) total parenteral nutrition (TPN) recommended for 7–10 days preoperatively.

225. *Factors responsible for intractability in PUD:* (a) penetration (the most common, in 50% of patients coming to surgery for intractability); (b) pyloric obstruction; (c) pyloric channel and postbulbar ulcers; (d) Z-E; (e) ulcerogenic drugs; and (f) smoking.

226. *Billroth I (gastroduodenostomy)* has been abandoned because of the high recurrence rate.

227. *Pancreatitis* is a potential complication of any operation that includes resection of the distal stomach and is related to trauma at the time of resection.

228. *Vagotomy* removes vagal stimulation on the parietal cells and reduces sensitivity of parietal cells to gastrin.

229. *The more selective the vagotomy*, the fewer the postoperative problems (diarrhea and gastric stasis).

230. *Superselective vagotomy* (also known as *parietal cell vagotomy* or *proximal gastric vagotomy*): (a) does not require a drainage procedure because antral motor function is retained; (b) is uncommonly associated with postoperative dumping and diarrhea (approximately 5%); and (c) is the operative procedure of choice for DU, but the recurrence rate is still unknown (2–10% according to preliminary observations).

231. Multiple surgical procedures are being used for the treatment of GU. The most common is *gastric resection*, including the resection of the ulcer, with or without vagotomy.

232. *A relatively new operation for GU* includes parietal cell vagotomy, no drainage procedure, and wedge resection of the ulcer. This procedure reduces acid secretion, maintains good gastric emptying, provides the entire ulcer for pathological examination, and does not facilitate duodenal reflux. Frequency of recurrence is unknown.

233. *Surgical options in GU* when the ulcer is in the fundus near the E – G junction include (a) Kelling–Madlender operation (biopsy of the ulcer and distal gastric resection, leaving the ulcer in place); and (b) vagotomy and antrectomy or drainage and biopsy or complete excision of the ulcer.

234. *Surgical options in bleeding ulcer (GU or DU)* include (a) vagotomy and oversew of the bleeding ulcer and pyloroplasty (low mortality, high recurrence rate of bleeding); and (b) vagotomy and antrectomy (15% mortality but low recurrence rate).

235. *Surgical approach in perforation*: (a) DU: closure with omental patch and parietal cell vagotomy; (b) benign GU: distal partial gastrectomy with or without vagotomy; when the patient is unstable, the ulcer should be biopsied and closed with an omental patch with no definitive surgery; and (c) malignant GU: resection should be attempted at the time of perforation if possible.

236. *Incidence of postoperative recurrent ulcer*: (a) post-Billroth II, 30–35%; (b) postproximal gastric vagotomy, 7–10%; (c) posttruncal vagotomy and drainage, 7–10%; (d) postsubtotal gastrectomy, 2–6%; and (e) posttruncal vagotomy and antrectomy, 1%.

237. *Causes of postoperative recurrent ulcer* include (a) incomplete vagotomy; (b) Z-E; (c) retained antrum; (d) ulcerogenic drugs; and (e) ulcer in surgical suture.

238. *Recurrent ulcer after surgery may present as* abdominal pain, bleeding, obstruction, perforation, gastrojejunocolic fistula (diarrhea, weight loss, and feculent breath or vomiting are the symptoms of the latter). There is a tendency to have symptoms similar to those caused by the preoperative ulcer.

239. The current view is that most recurrent *postoperative ulcers* respond to H_2-blockers; however, sometimes a prophylactic dose will be necessary on a continuous basis.

240. In anastomotic (stomal) ulcer, the pain is often periumbilical.

241. As many as two-thirds of *jejunal postoperative ulcers* will bleed; 5% will perforate.

242. *Achlorhydria* after surgery for PUD may lead to the presence of bacteria in the stomach, a predisposing factor for carcinogenesis.

243. *Superficial gastritis,* which may develop into *atrophic gastritis,* occurs after any form of partial gastrectomy. It is caused by reflux of bile and may be symptomless or present with abdominal pain unrelieved by food. Treatment of symptomatic patients is surgical—Roux-en-Y transposition of the afferent loop, to permit entry of bile and pancreatic juices into the jejunum 45 cm below the gastrojejunal anastomosis.

244. In adults, *relative lactose intolerance* may develop after ulcer surgery; this is the result of bypassing the lactase-rich duodenum.

245. Symptoms of *early dumping* (15–30 min after the meal): anxiety, weakness, dizziness, tachycardia, pounding pulse, sweating, flushing, abdominal cramps, and diarrhea.

246. Symptoms of *late dumping* (80–120 min after the meal) simulate the clinical manifestations of hypoglycemia.

247. *Management of early dumping*: (a) a piece of dry toast or cracker 15–20 min before the main meal; (b) frequent small meals with no fluid; (c) lying down after meals (delays emptying into jejunum); and (d) atropine and cyproheptadine, worth a try.

248. *Late dumping* is ascribed to hypoglycemia, is rare, and may be prevented by frequent meals or minimized by a high-protein, high-fat, low-carbohydrate diet.

249. *Afferent loop obstruction* (a) is rare; (b) causes severe vomiting and abdominal pain 10–20 min after meals when biliary and pancreatic secretions are maximal; and (c) is relieved by vomiting when drainage of the partially obstructed loop improves.

250. *Diarrhea after ulcer surgery*: (a) is due to rapid emptying of hypertonic fluid from the stomach, which overwhelms small intestinal absorptive capacity; (b) usually occurs 1–2 hr after meals; (c) is drastically reduced in incidence by parietal cell vagotomy.

251. *Steatorrhea after ulcer surgery* involving partial gastrectomy should suggest gastrojejunocolic fistula from jejunal ulcer or bacterial overgrowth (BOG) (see Chapter 3).

252. *Anemia after ulcer surgery* may be caused by (a) iron deficiency (bleeding from gastritis, inadequate intake of food from fear of pain); (b) B_{12} deficiency (consumed by BOG); and (c) folate deficiency (consumed by BOG and inadequate intake).

253. *Osteoporosis and osteomalacia after ulcer surgery*: (a) occur in 5–15% of patients after 6 years and more from surgery; (b) are caused by inadequate intake of calcium and vitamin D and by a selective defect in absorption; and (c) are less prevalent after vagotomy compared with Billroth surgery.

254. Inactive pulmonary tuberculosis may reactivate after gastrectomy. Vagotomy with no resection should be preferred in patients with previous TB.

255. Increased prevalence of gallstones has been reported after partial gastrectomy.

3
The Small and Large Intestine

1. The *jejunum* has been defined rather arbitrarily as the proximal two-fifths of the small intestine.

2. Anatomical differences between the proximal jejunum and the distal ileum are as follows: (a) the diameter of the jejunum is about twice that of the distal ileum; (b) the jejunal wall is thicker; (c) the jejunum has more plicae circularis; (d) the distal ileum has more Peyer's patches; and (e) the mesentery contains more fat in the distal ileum.

3. The surface area of the microscopic lining of the small bowel is far greater than the exterior muscle layer. This is due to the *villi* and the *brush border*. The latter is composed of multiple *microvilli* covered by *glycocalyx*, which contains many of the digestive enzymes.

4. *Brunner's glands* (a) are located mainly in the duodenal bulb and proximal duodenum; and (b) secrete mucus and HCO_3 to protect from acid.

5. The *intestinal villi* are tallest in the distal duodenum and proximal

jejunum and become progressively shorter toward the ileocecal valve.

6. The cells in the *crypt epithelium* of the small intestine are (a) *Paneth* cells, located in the base of the crypt (contain eosinophilic granules); (b) *goblet* cells (contain mucous granules); (c) *undifferentiated* cells (the most abundant); and (d) *endocrine* cells (contain secretory granules).

7. The cells in the epithelium that cover the intestinal villi are (a) *absorptive* cells (the luminal membrane of these cells forms the microvilli); (b) *goblet* cells; and (c) a few *endocrine* cells.

8. The functions of Paneth and undifferentiated cells are unknown.

9. The crypt epithelium contains at least 10 types of endocrine cells which secrete *gastrin, secretin, cholecystokinin (CCK), somatostatin, enteroglucagon,* motilin, neurotensin, GIP, VIP, and serotonin.

10. *M cells* are specialized epithelial cells overlying lymphoid follicles in Peyer's patches in the ileum. The name is derived from the thin membranous separation formed by the apical cytoplasm between the intestinal lumen and underlying lymphocytes and macrophages. These specialized cells probably provide a specific route for antigen uptake into the intestinal lymphoid system.

11. Unlike the jejunum and ileum, which have *mesentery* through their entire length, only the transverse and sigmoid segments of the colon have a mesentery.

12. *The rectum* begins at the termination of the pelvic mesocolon. The terminal 3-cm segment of the rectum is the anus (or anal canal). The rectum has no serosal layer, as it is outside the peritoneal space.

13. *Houston valves* are shelflike folds in the rectal mucosa, usually two on the left and one on the right.

14. *Blumer's shelf* is a firm, indurated ridgelike deformity felt on rectal examination when a tumor impinges on the anterior wall of the rectum.

15. The colonic mucosa contains no villi, but there are crypts (up to 0.7 mm deep) extending from the muscularis mucosa to the surface.

16. Cells in the *deeper half of colonic crypts* include (a) *proliferating undifferentiated* cells; (b) *mucus – secreting goblet* cells; and (c) at least six types of *endocrine* cells. Cells in the *superficial half of the crypt* include (a) *differentiating* absorptive cells; (b) *goblet* cells; and (c) a few *endocrine* cells.

17. The time from cell birth at the depth of the crypt to cell loss at the tip of the villi is (a) 5–7 days in the duodenum; (b) 4–5 days in the ileum; and (c) 4–6 days in the colon.

18. *Blood supply to the intestine*: (a) the superior mesenteric artery (SMA) supplies the jejunum, ileum, ascending colon, hepatic flexure, and proximal part of the transverse colon through its ileocolic, right colic, and middle colic branches; the jejunum and ileum are nourished by smaller intestinal branches of the SMA, and all the intestinal branches form a series of three or four arcades before entering the wall of the intestine as the arteriae rectae (the latter are end arteries); (b) the inferior mesenteric artery (IMA) supplies the distal transverse colon, the descending and sigmoid colon, and the proximal portions of the rectum through its left colic branch, two or three sigmoidal arteries, and a superior rectal artery; and (c) the lower parts of the rectum are supplied by the middle and inferior rectal arteries, which are branches of the hypogastric artery (itself a branch of the internal iliac artery).

19. *Major anastomoses in intestinal blood supply*: (a) the superior pancreaticoduodenal artery (a branch of the hepatic artery) anastomoses with the inferior pancreaticoduodenal artery (a branch of SMA) in the duodenum in the region of the head of the pancreas;

(b) the ileocolic artery anastomoses with the continuation of the main trunk of the SMA in the vicinity of the cecum; (c) the left colic artery (a branch of IMA) may connect with the middle colic artery (a branch of SMA) through the arch of Riolan, also known as the meandering mesenteric artery; and (d) the adjacent branches of the sigmoid, left colic, middle colic, right colic, and ileocolic arteries form an arterial channel that parallels the large intestine along its mesenteric aspect. (This channel is called the marginal artery of Drummond, and it gives rise to the arteriae rectae, which enter the wall of the colon.)

20. *Venous circulation of the intestine*: veins parallel arteries in the smaller branches and along portions of the main mesenteric trunks. The superior mesenteric vein joins the splenic vein to form the portal vein. The inferior mesenteric vein usually drains into the splenic vein.

21. *Functions of the small intestine*: (a) absorption; (b) secretion; and (c) motility.

22. *Somatostatin* is capable of inhibiting absorption, secretion, motility, and, to some extent, splanchnic circulation.

23. *Duplications* are spherical or tubular cysts attached to a portion of the GI tract. They occur mainly in the ileum and can cause obstruction.

24. *Meckel's diverticle*: (a) is a remnant of the vitelline duct; (b) is the most frequent congenital anomaly of the intestinal tract (0.3–3% in autopsy reports); (c) is mostly asymptomatic but may lead to volvulus, intussusception, peptic ulcer in the adjacent ileal mucosa (when it contains ectopic gastric mucosa), bleeding, and perforation; (d) can be demonstrated by enteroclysis or, when it contains gastric mucosa, by technetium scan; and (e) according to current view, should not be removed, when found incidentally in an asymptomatic patient.

25. *Types of peristaltic waves in the small intestine* include (a) *type 1*: segmental contractions of circular muscle, 10–12/min, 2–6 sec in duration, facilitate absorption but do not produce forward motion; (b) *type 2*: slow, strong waves, rarely seen in normal small bowel, similar to type 1 but longer (10 sec to 8 min) and occur less regularly; (c) *type 3*: superimposed on type 1, narrow the lumen to sweep the intestinal contents forward; and (d) *type 4*: occur only in ileostomy patients with a rise in pressure and tone and simultaneous effacement of type 1 waves.

26. *Migrating motor complex (MMC)*: (a) it is a wave that occurs every 84–112 min in the fasting state that migrates 6–8 cm/min from the duodenum to the terminal ileum; (b) it is the "intestinal housekeeper" that moves interdigestive contents down the small intestine, preventing stagnation and bacterial growth; (c) its initiation closely correlates with peak blood levels of motilin; and (d) it is terminated by food.

27. *Scleroderma* and *intestinal pseudoobstruction* are motility disorders wherein stasis leads to bacterial overgrowth (BOG) and subsequent malabsorption.

28. *Colonic motility*: (a) contractions originating in the transverse and ascending colon move toward the cecum more often than distally; (b) absorption is facilitated by this retrograde propagation; (c) nonpropulsive segmental movements have been demonstrated; and (d) mass propulsion is seen in 6% of subjects during fasting.

29. Increased colonic motility is caused by gastrin and CCK, while secretin and glucagon decrease motility.

30. In *diverticulosis* of the colon, slow-wave activity is increased to 18 cycles/min and the intraluminal pressure is elevated.

31. In *diabetes mellitus*, constipation (an abnormality of colonic motility) is more common than diarrhea (an abnormality of small intestinal motility).

32. *Metoclopramide* has been shown to be of benefit in constipation of diabetic neuropathy.

33. *Cholinergic agents* stimulate colonic contractility and are effective in scleroderma, intestinal pseudoobstruction, and constipation of diabetic neuropathy.

34. Distention of the rectum leads to relaxation of the internal anal sphincter and to contraction of the external anal sphincter.

35. *Phenytoin* (Dilantin) and *sulfasalazine* decrease folic acid absorption in humans.

36. Malabsorption leads to *folic acid deficiency* more rapidly than does dietary deficiency alone because there is an enterohepatic circulation for folic acid that adds 100 μg of this metabolite daily to the average daily consumption of 200–400 μg. Tissue stores are relatively small—5 mg.

37. The *cobalamin* produced by bacteria in the colon is not absorbed.

38. *Cobalamin* in the stomach binds to R proteins. The cobalamin–R protein complex leaves the stomach along with free IF. In the upper small intestine, pancreatic proteases hydrolyze the R protein, thereby liberating free cobalamin, which now binds to IF. The intrinsic factor–cobalamin complex in dimeric form traverses the small bowel, reaching its site of absorption in the distal ileum.

39. *Cobalamin deficiency* is very uncommon in patients with pancreatic insufficiency probably because under these circumstances enough cobalamin binds to IF, even in the presence of intact R proteins.

40. The daily consumption of cobalamin (1 μg) is very small compared with the size of its stores in the liver (5000 μg). Thus, cobalamin deficiency in the diet slowly leads to clinical deficiency but, when malabsorption is present, deficiency develops more rapidly as a result of losses from the enterohepatic circulation.

41. *Iron* is absorbed mainly in the duodenum.

42. Red blood cells (RBCs) contain most of the body iron stores (more than the liver and the spleen).

43. *Micelles* contain fatty acids, monoglycerides, fat-soluble vitamins (A, D, E, and K), bile salts, cholesterol, and phospholipids.

44. *Critical micellar concentration (CMC)* is the intraluminal concentration of bile salts required for the formation of mixed micelles. It is usually 2–5 mM.

45. *Chylomicrons* contain triglycerides (90%), cholesterol ester (1%), free cholesterol (1%), phospholipid (7%), and apoprotein (1%).

46. *Medium-chain triglycerides (MCT)*: (a) are triglycerides with a side chain length of 8–10 carbons (as opposed to 16–18 in long-chain triglycerides); (b) are hydrolyzed by lipase in the lumen of the gut more rapidly than are long-chain triglycerides; (c) are water soluble and rapidly absorbed (there is no need for bile salts and micelle formation); (d) are absorbed straight into the portal system, bypassing the lymphatics; and (e) supply 7 cal/g.

47. *Starch* is rapidly digested in the duodenum by large amounts of secreted pancreatic amylase.

48. *Disaccharides* are absorbed in the proximal small intestine. *Oligosaccharides* and *peptides* are absorbed in the ileum.

49. *Pepsin* is not essential for protein digestion, as there is an overabundance of pancreatic proteases in the duodenum, jejunum, and proximal ileum.

50. Intestinal absorption of ingested *protein* is mainly through absorption of amino acids, but it has a mechanism that absorbs dipeptides and tripeptides, especially those containing a glycine or a proline residue.

51. In an infant less than 1 week old, some *proteins* can be absorbed without hydrolysis.

52. *Resection* of up to 40% of the *small bowel* is usually well tolerated if the duodenum, the proximal jejunum, the distal half of the ileum, and the ileocecal valve are spared. Resection of 50% or more of the small bowel usually results in malabsorption. Resection of 70% is life threatening. Preservation of the ileocecal valve is important because it prolongs transit time and prevents bacterial overgrowth in the small intestine.

53. *Gastrin hypersecretion* is present in 50% of patients after extensive *small bowel resection* and may lead to peptic ulcer disease. The cause is unknown.

54. *Resection (or bypassing) of the duodenum* may lead to deficiency of *iron, folate,* and *calcium* (osteomalacia).

55. *Resection of the distal ileum* may lead to diarrhea and steatorrhea due to disruption of the enterohepatic circulation of bile salts.

56. If less than 100 cm of the distal ileum is resected, there is *cholerrheic diarrhea* but no significant steatorrhea. The diarrhea is caused by bile salts that reach the colon and impair water and ion absorption and stimulate secretion, but the liver is able to compensate for the reduced absorption of bile salts and *steatorrhea* is not present.

57. *Cholestyramine* is effective in *cholerrheic diarrhea* when it prevents the entry of excessive amounts of bile salts to the colon by binding bile salts in the ileum. Cholestyramine will aggravate *steatorrheic diarrhea* by further depleting the available bile salt pool.

58. Differentiation of *cholerrheic* from *steatorrheic diarrhea* is possible by measuring stool fat content (high only in the latter) or vitamin B_{12} absorptive capacity (better in the former), or with a therapeutic trial with cholestyramine.

59. According to recent studies, the concentration of stool fat is higher in steatorrhea of pancreatic insufficiency when compared with steatorrhea of other causes.

60. *Management of short bowel syndrome,* after extensive resection of small intestine, includes (a) total parenteral nutrition (TPN); (b) antidiarrheal agents (Lomotil, Imodium, tincture of opium, codeine, anticholinergics); (c) oral feeding, started as soon as possible (MCT, amino acids, simple sugars at the beginning); (d) antimicrobial agents for bacterial overgrowth; (e) H_2-blockers for gastric hypersecretion; and (f) B_{12} after extensive ileal resection.

61. In *short bowel syndrome* hyperoxaluria may develop when the colon is intact due to excessive colonic absorption of oxalate. Possible mechanisms: (a) excessive quantities of fatty acids in the gut form soaps with calcium, reducing its availability for formation of insoluble calcium oxalate, leading to persistence of soluble and absorbable oxalate in the colon; and (b) the presence of bile salts and fatty acids in the colon increases its permeability to oxalate. The management of hyperoxaluria (which may develop by the same mechanism in any severe steatorrhea with intact colon) includes administration of a low-oxalate, high-calcium diet and maintenance of high urinary volume.

62. In *short bowel syndrome* lactic acidosis may develop due to generation of *d*-lactate by colonic anaerobic bacteria exposed to high concentrations of unabsorbed carbohydrates.

63. The normal osmolarity of the stool is about 300 mmol/liter. It equals the sum of sodium and potassium stool concentration multiplied by 2 + a gap of 30–40 mmol/liter. In osmotic diarrhea (most common after eating lactose in lactase deficiency), the gap may increase to around 100 mmol/liter.

64. The normal colon is capable of absorbing up to 5000 ml water, 800 mEq sodium, and 44 mEq potassium daily. Larger loads lead to diarrhea.

65. *High-volume diarrhea,* 1000–2000 ml/day, relieved by fasting is most commonly an osmotic diarrhea of exogenous origin (lactase deficiency).

66. *High-volume diarrhea* unrelieved by fasting is usually of *endog-*

enous origin—stimulation of secretory processes of the small intestine as in cholera or carcinoid syndrome.

67. *Small-volume diarrhea* is characteristic of steatorrhea and colonic diseases.

68. The stimulation of secretion in the *secretory diarrhea* induced by unabsorbed fatty acids will disappear when the patient stops taking excessive fat in the diet.

69. Mechanisms of action of various *antidiarrheal agents*: (a) *opiates* (Lomotil, Imodium, codeine) have an antimotility action and a stimulatory effect on water and electrolyte absorption; (b) *alpha-adrenergic agonists*, such as clonidine, stimulate sodium and chloride absorption; (c) somatostatin stimulates water and electrolyte absorption; (d) chlorpromazine interrupts intracellular events that are probably calcium mediated, and it may decrease diarrhea; and (e) prostaglandin synthetase inhibitors decrease water and electrolyte secretion.

70. *Melanosis coli* usually disappears within 3–6 months after discontinuation of anthracene laxatives.

71. *Irritable bowel syndrome (IBS)* is a motility disorder. Whereas the normal frequency of colonic slow waves is 6 cycles/min, in IBS it is 3 cycles/min in at least 40% of cases and postprandial colonic hypermotility is delayed for 70–100 min. High-amplitude pressure waves and segmental contractions are common.

72. *Possible manifestations of IBS*: (a) most patients have painful spastic abdominal discomfort with *constipation* or *diarrhea*, whereas a few have painless diarrhea; (b) spasm may lead to "pencil-thin," "ribbonlike," or "marblelike" stool; (c) abdominal pain is often stimulated by food, relieved by defecation, does not awaken the patient at night, is diffuse or localized to left lower quadrant (LLQ); (d) diarrhea often consists of small volumes of stool; (e) extreme urgency or tenesmus are typical; (f) patients complain of belching and flatus (but increased amounts of gas have not been documented); (g) mucus in the stool is uncommon but characteristic; and (h) dysmenorrhea, urinary frequency, dyspareunia, and headache are common.

73. Possible *findings on physical examination in IBS*: (a) the patient is unable to locate the pain precisely; (b) the colon is tender to palpation, the cecum is often palpable; and (c) abdominal tenderness often disappears on persistent pressure.

74. On *sigmoidoscopy in IBS*: (a) a spastic contraction may be seen and may prevent passage of the instrument beyond 10–12 cm; (b) the procedure is painful; (c) air insufflation may reproduce the symptoms; and (d) mucus may be present, but the mucosa should be free of ulcers, bleeding, friability, and masses.

75. *Diagnostic studies that should be performed before entertaining the diagnosis of IBS* are: CBC; stool for ova and parasites (including *Giardia* and *amebae*); stool for occult blood; sigmoidoscopy; barium enema; a trial of a lactose-free diet for 3 weeks in patients with distention, bloating, or diarrhea; upper GI series when dyspeptic symptoms are present; and small bowel series when diarrhea or symptoms suggestive of obstruction are present.

76. *Management of IBS*: (a) a high-fiber diet (12–16 g unprocessed bran daily); (b) psyllium preparations such as Metamucil at mealtime; (c) anticholinergics (such as Bentyl or Probanthine) 30–45 min before meals; (d) low doses of cholestyramine (2 g with each meal) are helpful at times; (e) antidepressants such as amitriptyline 25 mg qid have been found to be more effective than tranquilizers; (f) when constipation predominates a diet rich in cooked fruits, vegetables, and liquids and daily physical exercise are effective and the patient should refrain from laxatives; and (g) if diarrhea predominates, the patient should avoid cooked and uncooked fruits and vegetables or alcohol and antidiarrheal agents should be administered in a low dose (Lomotil, Imodium, or codeine).

77. *Dietary fiber* is the plant material in the diet that is resistant to digestion in the gut.

78. The average American eats 8–11 g fiber per day and the average Briton 4–8 g, while vegetarians consume 12–24 g/day.

79. The *effects of fiber* are (a) to shorten intestinal transit time; (b) to increase stool volume and to act as osmotic cathartics by conversion of the fiber to water and short-chain fatty acids; and (c) to further increase the bulk of the stool by the action of cellulose (a major constituent of fiber) to absorb water.

80. Normally 400–1500 cc of flatus is being passed daily, of which 50% is nitrogen, 40% is carbon dioxide, and the remainder is composed of hydrogen, methane, and very small amounts of oxygen. The amount and proportion of gases vary widely depending on the amount swallowed, the diet, and the type of intestinal bacteria.

81. *Management of excessive intestinal gas* is rarely satisfactory. Patients should be advised to eat slowly and to avoid chewing gum, carbonated beverages, artificial sweeteners, legumes, and foods of the cabbage family. Therapeutic agents that may be of benefit are simethicone, antacids, antibiotics, activated charcoal, pancreatic enzymes, and metoclopramide. Physical exercise, discontinuation of smoking, and a heating pad to the abdomen should be tried.

82. *Proctalgia fugax* (a) is a severe, sudden spasmodic pain deep in the rectum; (b) lasts from 20 sec to a few minutes; (c) is common at night; (d) occurs in about 20% of the population; and (e) may be relieved by firm upper pressure on the anus.

83. *Small bowel diverticles* are more common in the proximal than in the distal small intestine. Intermittent small-volume bleeding is the most common complication.

84. *Colonic diverticulosis* occurs in 10% of people in developed countries, is rare before the age of 40, and increases in prevalence from

5% in the fifth decade to 50% in the ninth decade. Only 20% of patients with diverticles have symptoms.

85. In *simple massed diverticulosis*, there are multiple diverticles and the musculature of the colonic wall is weakened. In *spastic colon diverticulosis*, there are few diverticles and muscular hypertrophy.

86. *Spastic colon diverticulosis* may be the result of IBS.

87. In *scleroderma*, there are *wide-mouthed diverticles* in the colon.

88. Uncomplicated diverticulosis is usually an asymptomatic condition. Possible rare symptoms are (a) LLQ pain, which may be aggravated by food and relieved by passing stool or flatus; and (b) painless rectal bleeding.

89. *Diverticular bleeding* (a) is located in the right colon in 70% of cases; (b) usually begins in a single diverticle, which in 80% of cases is not inflamed; (c) may be massive and may last hours to days intermittently or continuously; (d) stops spontaneously in 80% of cases; (e) recurs within days to years in 20–25% of cases.

90. *Management of a suspected diverticular bleeding* includes (a) the passage of nasogastric tube and aspiration of the stomach to exclude upper GI source; (b) proctosigmoidoscopy to rule out bleeding lesions in the lower GI tract; (c) radionuclide imaging with [^{99m}Tc]-sulfur colloid or RBCs to define the approximate location of active bleeding; (d) arteriography, if bleeding continues, the inferior mesenteric artery should be entered first and then the SMA; (e) a trial of intraarterial vasopressin or transcatheter arterial embolization of the bleeding vessel, if bleeding continues; (f) if that fails segmental resection of the portion of the colon containing the bleeding diverticle should be performed.

91. *Barium enema* can preclude the performance of a satisfactory angiographic study for 1–7 days.

92. In 10–20% of patients with diverticulosis diverticulitis will develop. It is more common in patients with numerous diverticles that are widely distributed in the colon, that appear at an early age, or that have been known to be present for a decade or two. In most cases, only one diverticle, which is commonly located in the sigmoid colon, is involved in the inflammatory process.

93. *Pain* and *fever* are the most common presenting symptoms of diverticulitis.

94. In *diverticulitis*, perforation with the development of paracolic abscesses or fistulas to adjacent organs (bladder, ureter, vagina, small bowel, skin) is common, but free perforation is rare.

95. The *diagnostic approach to diverticulitis* includes (a) a gentle proctosigmoidoscopy with minimal bowel preparation and no air insufflation to reveal the presence of diverticles, to assess whether other inflammatory disorders are present, and to exclude obstruction from carcinoma; (b) plain films of the abdomen, to help assess the degree of ileus and reveal free air in the rare case of free perforation; (c) a carefully performed barium enema, recommended by most authors to demonstrate a paracolic mass, a fistula, or a narrowed segment; (d) intravenous pyelography (IVP) or cystoscopy, which may be helpful in patients with urinary tract involvement.

96. *Diverticulitis* and *Crohn's disease* can occur simultaneously in the same patient, posing a difficult differential diagnosis. Diverticulitis and ulcerative colitis rarely coexist in the same patient.

97. When spastic abdominal pain is ascribed to *diverticulosis*, bran (2 teaspoons of unprocessed bran tid) may be helpful in relieving spasm and in "keeping the lumen open."

98. *Management of diverticulitis* includes (a) bed rest; (b) NPO (nasogastric tube if ileus is present); and (c) administration of antibiotic agents only if fever, ileus, or signs of pericolic abscess are present.

99. In *diverticulitis* 70–80% of patients respond to conservative treatment, and two-thirds of these patients will not have another attack requiring hospitalization. In 15–30% of patients with diverticulitis, surgery will be required.

100. *Hirschprung's disease (congenital megacolon)* (a) occurs in 1 of 5000 live births; (b) has a male to female ratio of 3.8:1; (c) is familial in 8% of patients; (d) has an association with Down's syndrome that is ten times more than the expected incidence; (e) is characterized by the absence of ganglion cells from the submucosal and intramuscular plexuses, and abnormal hypertrophied nerve fibers may be present; and (f) in the "short segment" form, is limited to the anus or rectum (relatively uncommon); in 75% of patients, the disease involves the rectum and lower sigmoid; longer segments of the colon or even the small intestine may be involved.

101. In *Hirschprung's disease* the internal anal sphincter fails to relax following rectal distention and the rectal wall is "stiff."

102. *Symptoms of Hirschprung's disease* are variable—the disorder can be asymptomatic, there can be recurrent episodes of bowel obstruction, enterocolitis early in infancy carries a poor prognosis, and perforation or stercoral ulcers are occasional manifestations.

103. Rectal biopsy and barium enema are required to confirm the *diagnosis of Hirschprung's disease*—the former to verify the anatomic lesion and the latter to define its extent. If no ganglion cells are seen on deep mucosal biospy taken through a sigmoidoscope, a full-thickness surgical biopsy should be obtained.

104. *Management of Hirschprung's disease* includes (a) an early colostomy, which serves to prevent the development of enterocolitis and to delay the performance of definitive surgery until growth is attained; and (b) a pull-through procedure.

105. *Encopresis (fecal soiling)* is typical of *idiopathic megacolon* and is absent in patients with Hirschprung's disease.

106. *Volvulus of the colon* can occur in the cecum or in the sigmoid.

The former is associated with congenital abnormalities, such as situs inversus, and the latter with constipation, high-fiber diets, or other factors that lead to a large, dilated sigmoid.

107. *Pneumatosis cystoides intestinalis* is composed of multiple air-filled cysts in the submucosa of the colon caused by a fulminant infectious or ischemic process. It has been reported in perforated peptic ulcer, scleroderma, and COPD. It is usually asymptomatic but may cause obstruction or volvulus. Inhalation of 55–75% O_2 reduces the size of the cysts.

108. In *acute infectious diarrhea* the colonic flora become less anaerobic because of the rapid transit. The pathogen itself dominates the intestinal flora.

109. *Tenesmus* occurring in infectious diarrhea implicates colonic involvement and may be present in infections with *Shigella, Campylobacter,* and invasive *E. coli.*

110. *Salmonella* and *Yersinia* involve principally the lower small bowel but may invade the colon as well.

111. Toxigenic *E. coli, Vibrio cholera,* and *Giardia* are small bowel pathogens—WBCs or RBCs are not found in the stool in infections caused by these organisms.

112. Bacteria may provoke *acute diarrhea* by (a) infiltration of colonic mucosa to produce a dysenterylike process (Shigellosis); (b) invasion of the lumen of the relatively sterile small bowel to provoke a choleralike syndrome with massive fluid loss (enteropathogenic *E. coli*); and (c) deconjugation of bile salts, which leads to steatorrhea and hydroxylation of fatty acids.

113. In *cholera* (a) the origin of fluid loss is in the upper small intestine, where the enterotoxin has its greatest activity; (b) there are no white blood cells on stool smear and there is no bacteremia—it is an enterotoxicogenic diarrhea; (c) small intestinal epithelium does not demonstrate histologic changes; (d) the stool is isotonic with the plasma but there is an excessive loss of *potassium* and *bicarbonate*, producing hypokalemic acidosis; (e) management includes isotonic fluids, KCl, bicarbonate, tetracyclines, 40 mg/kg for 2 days; (f) close contacts should be given tetracycline 1 g/day for 5 days as prophylaxis; and (g) the carrier state is uncommon but, when it occurs, commonly involves the gallbladder.

114. In *Shigellosis* (a) the serotype *S. dysenteriae* produces the severest form of dysentery and *S. sonnei* produces the mildest disease; (b) the most common clinical findings are *lower abdominal pain* and *diarrhea* with fever present in 40% of patients and typical dysentery stool (with blood and mucus) present in one third; (c) intestinal complications include perforation and protein loss, and extraintestinal complications are coryza, cough, meningismus, convulsions, rash, hemolytic-uremic syndrome, thrombocytopenia, and arthritis of large joints; (d) carriers have been identified, but they are uncommon; (e) carriers are susceptible to intermittent attacks of the disease, in contrast to *Salmonella* carriers (see below); (f) opiates are contraindicated, as they prolong the disease and may lead to megacolon; (g) antimicrobial agents (ampicillin for 5 days or trimethoprim-sulfamethoxazole or tetracyclines for resistant strains) should be administered only when symptoms are severe; and (h) carriers should receive trimethoprim-sulfamethoxazole for 28 days.

115. In clinical syndromes caused by *Salmonella* (a) gastroenteritis is noted in 70% of salmonella infections; (b) bacteremia occurs in 10%; (c) "enteric fever" or "typhoidal type" is seen in all typhoidal strains and in 8% of other salmonella infections; (d) localized infections (bones, joints, and meninges) occur in about 5%; and (e) the patient may be an asymptomatic carrier.

116. *Salmonella colitis* has been reported in a small minority of patients. In these patients diarrhea is prolonged compared with salmonella without colitis.

117. *Management of salmonella gastroenteritis:* (a) No antibiotic therapy should be given in uncomplicated salmonella gastroenteritis; (b) antibiotic agents should be administered in salmonella gastroenteritis when lymphoproliferative disorders or prosthetic valves or other implanted foreign bodies are present or in babies and the elderly, and in septicemia; and (c) the drugs of choice are ampicillin or trimethoprim-sulfamethoxazole for 10–14 days.

118. In *typhoid fever:* (a) intestinal bleeding occurs in about 7% of patients; (b) intestinal perforation is experienced by approximately 3% and occurs most commonly in the terminal ileum; and (c) intestinal hemorrhage and perforation may occur in the same patient, with both most apt to occur during the third week and convalescence and not closely related to the severity of the disease.

119. In *typhoid fever* relapses are common 8–10 days after cessation of antimicrobial therapy and consist of a reenactment of the major manifestations.

120. In *typhoid fever* 50% of patients excrete the organism in the feces after 6 weeks, 5–10% after 3 months, and 1–3% after 1 year.

121. *Management of typhoid fever:* (a) Chloramphenicol is the standard therapy and should be administered for 2 weeks; (b) amoxicillin, ampicillin, and cotrimoxazole have been used successfully as alternative modes of therapy; (c) corticosteroids should be administered to patients with severe toxemia; (d) intestinal perforation is managed surgically; (e) salicylates should be avoided; (f) a relapse should be treated with the same antimicrobial agent that had been given for the first attack; (g) ampicillin, 6 g/day for 6 weeks, is recommended for the chronic carrier who has been discharging *S. typhi* for longer than 1 year; (h) cholecystectomy is recommended only for those whose profession is incompatible with the typhoid carrier state (food handlers and health care providers) if reappearance of the carrier state occurs following ampicillin therapy; and (i) a typhoid vaccine that affords 70% protection is recommended for travelers to endemic regions.

122. *Campylobacter fetus* ss. *jejuni*: (a) This is probably the most common cause of bacterial diarrhea; (b) it has an incubation period of 24–72 hr but may extend up to 10 days; (c) clinical manifestations are variable and run from frank dysentery with diarrhea, fever, abdominal pain, and bloody stools to asymptomatic excretion; (d) clinical illness may last for 1–2 weeks; (e) relapses occur in 25% of patients; (f) erythromycin, 1–2 g/day for 1 week, is the preferred therapy.

123. The spectrum of clinical illnesses caused by *Yersinia enterocolitica*: (a) Enterocolitis occurs in children less than 5 years of age; (b) in children over 5 years of age ileitis and mesenteric adenitis have been described; (c) in adults yersinia is less common and may cause acute diarrhea, which may be followed by arthralgia, erythema nodosum, and erythema multiforme, a symptom complex associated with the HLA-B27 antigen; and (d) yersinia bacteremia may be seen in debilitated patients.

124. *Bacterial food poisoning* in the United States is caused by *Salmonella* (50%), *Staphylococcus aureus* (25%), *Clostridium perfringens* (11%), and *Shigella* (9%).

125. Specific *viral agents associated with diarrheal illness* consist of two main groups: rotavirus in children under 2 years of age and the Norwalk viruses that appear in epidemics attacking all age groups.

126. *Traveler's diarrhea*: (a) Symptoms usually occur 4–6 days after arrival and last for 2–4 days but may extend up to a few weeks; (b) fatigue, cramps, nausea, fever, and abdominal pain are commonly associated symptoms; (c) toxigenic *E. coli* is an important etiologic agent (probably responsible for 40–70% of cases); (d) 25–50% of American tourists to Mexico develop the disorder; (e) recommended therapy in addition to rehydration consists of bismuth subsalicylate, 30–60 ml tid for 3 days; and (f) bismuth subsalicylate, 60 ml qid, or doxycycline, 100 mg once a day, taken throughout the traveling period, has been successful in preventing traveler's diarrhea.

127. *In tuberculosis of the GI tract* (a) 50% of patients have no concomitant pulmonary disease; (b) in 85–90% of cases, the cecum is involved, but multiple areas of the bowel can be involved as well; (c) the clinical presentation is not specific and includes right lower quadrant pain, mass in the right lower quadrant, weight loss, low-grade fever, anorexia, diarrhea, or constipation; and (d) management includes a three-drug regimen for a period of 18 months and surgery for obstruction or fistulas that do not respond to conservative therapy.

128. *Reactive arthritis* may follow specific ulcerative enteritis such as that caused by *Yersinia enterocolitica, Campylobacter, Salmonella,* and *C. difficile.*

129. In *giardiasis* (a) most patients harboring the parasite are asymptomatic; (b) malabsorption may occur in children; (c) the parasite has been reported to cause traveler's diarrhea, mainly among tourists to the U.S.S.R., (d) an association occurs between the disease and the dysgammaglobulinemias; (e) the parasite is not found in the stool in at least 50% of patients, and the diagnosis is made by duodenal aspiration or small bowel biopsy; and (f) the recommended treatment is quinacrine, 100 mg tid for 7 days, or metronidazole, 250 mg tid for 7 days.

130. In *amebiasis* (a) the parasite infects the colon, with the cecum and ascending colon involved more frequently than the descending colon; (b) the pathologic lesions are flask-shaped ulcers with undermined edges; (c) many patients have only a mild diarrhea with some mucus, but others may have amebic dysentery simulating ulcerative colitis; (d) toxic megacolon is a possible complication of acute amebic colitis, and the administration of steroids in this setting is extremely hazardous; (e) the management of intestinal amebiasis includes diiodohydroxyquin (iodoquinol) or diloxanide furoate (Furamide) for asymptomatic intestinal infection, metronidazole, or paromomycin for moderate to severe intestinal disease; and (f) toxic megacolon that does not respond to conservative management or intestinal perforation is an indication for surgery.

131. *Normal microbial population of the alimentary tract*: stomach: $0-10^3$ (mainly aerobes); jejunum: $0-10^4$ (mainly aerobes); ileum: 10^5-10^8 (aerobes and anaerobes); and cecum: $10^{10}-10^{12}$ (anaerobes predominant).

132. *Bacterial overgrowth (BOG)* within the small intestine is known as the blind loop or stagnant loop syndrome and it may lead to malabsorption. It may occur following abdominal surgery, in structural abnormalities such as diverticles of the small intestine or Crohn's disease, and in motor abnormalities such as scleroderma or diabetic neuropathy. Achlorhydria may cause BOG, especially when combined with a motor or anatomic disturbance.

133. In *BOG* malabsorption is caused by abnormalities within the intraluminal environment (e.g., bacterial hydrolysis of conjugated bile salts) and from direct damage to the small bowel enterocytes.

134. In *BOG* malabsorption of vitamin B_{12} is caused by anaerobic bacteria which (a) utilize B_{12}; (b) bind intrinsic factor-B_{12} complex; and (c) probably produce analogues of B_{12} that compete with B_{12} for absorption.

135. In *BOG* serum folate levels may be high due to synthesis of folate by the microorganisms in the small bowel.

136. In *BOG* steatorrhea is caused by (a) deconjugation of bile salts by the microorganisms; (b) hydroxylation of fatty acids by the microorganism and inhibition of absorption by the metabolic products of this process; and (c) mucosal injury.

137. In *BOG* hypoproteinemia is caused by (a) exudative enteropathy; (b) mucosal injury; and (c) utilization of dietary protein by intestinal bacteria.

138. A definitive *diagnosis of BOG* is made by obtaining a cultured aspirate from the proximal small intestine under anaerobic conditions. The total concentration of bacteria generally exceeds 10^5 organisms per ml. Bacteroids, anaerobic lactobacilli, coliforms, and enterococci are all likely to be present.

139. *Management of BOG:* (a) surgical correction of the anatomic abnormality of the intestine, when feasible; (b) antimicrobial agents; for those who do not improve on tetracyclines within 1 week, metronidazole, clindamycin, or chloramphenicol should be tried; some patients require a 7- to 10-day course once in a few months, while others need more frequent courses; and (c) nutritional support by MCT, elimination of lactose from the diet, and administration of vitamin B_{12} injections and correction of other nutritional deficiencies (e.g., calcium, vitamin K).

140. In *Whipple's disease:* (a) clinical findings may include intestinal malabsorption, fever, skin pigmentation, anemia, lymphadenopathy, arthralgia and arthritis, pleuritis, pericarditis, endocarditis, and CNS symptoms; (b) the causative agent is probably a small rod-shaped bacillus that can be found infiltrating involved tissue; (c) cure is achieved with the administration of tetracyclines, but resistance has been reported and relapses do occur; penicillin is reported to be curative when resistance to tetracyclines is observed.

141. *Tropical sprue* is a chronic disease, endemic in the tropics, for which bacterial infection seems the most likely cause.

142. *Tropical sprue:* (a) Deficiency of both folate and vitamin B_{12} is characteristic of advanced disease; (b) in 50% of patients atrophic gastritis with achlorhydria is present; (c) the histologic changes are similar to the changes in celiac disease (see below) but less severe and with involvement of the ileum; and (d) treatment is with folate, vitamin B_{12} and tetracyclines.

143. *Celiac sprue* is a relatively common disease (prevalence is estimated at 0.03% of the general population). Its incidence is highest in northwestern Europe, about 85% of the patients are females, and there are two peaks of onset—the first in early infancy and the second in the fourth or fifth decade of life.

144. Characteristic lesion of the small intestinal mucosa in *celiac sprue*: (a) It has a flat mucosal surface with complete absence of normal intestinal villi; (b) there is a marked elongation of intestinal crypts; (c) the few absorptive cells that line the luminal surface are cuboidal or even squamous, but not columnar, with basophilic cytoplasm and loss of basal polarity of the nucleus; (d) the undifferentiated crypt cells are markedly increased in number; (e) the lamina propria is infiltrated with plasma cells and lymphocytes; and (f) the duodenum and jejunum, but not the ileum, are involved.

145. In *celiac sprue* (a) 80% of the patients are HLA-B8 and HLA-DW3 positive, compared with up to 20% in the general population; (b) first-order relatives of patients with celiac sprue show a 10% prevalence of latent celiac disease; and (c) most patients with dermatitis herpetiformis have latent celiac sprue, but the opposite is not true.

146. In *celiac sprue* (a) the natural history of untreated disease is one of intermittent exacerbations and remissions; (b) symptoms may be apparent in infancy when gluten is first ingested, diminish during adolescence, and reappear during the third and fourth decades; (c) the most common symptoms in extensive disease are diarrhea, flatulence, weight loss, and weakness; (d) abdominal pain is rarely seen; (e) pancreatic insufficiency occurs as a result of malnutrition and from impaired CCK and secretin release by the damaged duodenal mucosa; (f) the degree of steatorrhea correlates reasonably well with the severity and extent of the intestinal lesion; (g) metabolic bone disease and tetany may occur as a result of calcium and magnesium deficiency; and (h) high enteroglucagon levels have been found in untreated disease and reverted to normal upon successful therapy.

147. X-ray films of the small bowel after a barium meal in *celiac sprue* show (a) dilatation; (b) coarsening or obliteration of the mucosal folds; (c) fragmentation and flocculation of the barium; and (d) prolonged transit time.

148. *Management of celiac sprue*: (a) A strict gluten-free diet is mandatory; symptomatic improvement within 1 or 2 weeks is observed in most patients; recovery of the histologic lesion may be delayed for months or even for a few years; (b) prednisone (10–40 mg/day) should be tried in refractory patients; (c) some patients have primary or secondary lactase deficiency, and milk products should be removed from the diet; (d) replacement of vitamins and minerals should be instituted; and (e) after a period on gluten-free diet, some adults will be able to tolerate small amounts of gluten, but in children with celiac sprue it is recommended to continue with a gluten-free diet during the period of growth.

149. Possible reasons for lack of response to gluten-free diet in *suspected celiac sprue*: (a) poor adherence to the diet (most common); (b) intestinal lymphoma (see below); (c) collagenous sprue (see below); and (d) intestinal strictures and ulcers.

150. In *collagenous sprue* the mucosa is even thinner than in celiac sprue and a thick band of eosinophilic material appears under the epithelial cells. It is controversial whether collagenous sprue is a separate entity, but it is definitely characterized by its refractory nature to all forms of therapy.

151. *Eosinophilic gastroenteritis*: (a) There are three clinical syndromes: (i) predominant mucosal disease where *protein loss, anemia, and malabsorption* are prominent, (ii) predominant muscle layer disease where *pyloric and intestinal obstruction* are prominent, and (iii) predominant subserosal disease where *eosinophil-rich ascites* dominate the clinical picture; (b) most patients have elevated serum ·levels of IgG, eosinophilia (up to 80%), and history of some "food allergy"; (c) management includes steroids, from which most patients benefit; antihistamines have not proved of benefit and cromolyn sodium is still experimental at this writing.

152. *Pseudomembranous enterocolitis:* (a) The inflammation and necrosis of the bowel occur predominantly in the mucosa but may extend into the submucosa and rarely to deeper layers; (b) it is most commonly associated with the administration of antimicrobial agents, but poor blood perfusion may bring about a similar clinical and histologic picture; and (c) the lesions are in both the small and large bowel but are more prominent in the colon; at flexible sigmoidoscopy, pseudomembranes are seen in more than 90% of patients.

153. *Pseudomembranous enterocolitis* has been reported following the use of nearly all antimicrobial agents. Clindamycin and its parent compound lincomycin are implicated most often, but cephalosporin (oral and parenteral formulations) and ampicillin are also frequently involved.

154. Diarrhea is the most common symptom of *pseudomembranous enterocolitis.* About 60% of patients develop diarrhea while still on antimicrobial agents, while the others develop diarrhea within 4–6 weeks after discontinuation of antibiotics. The diarrhea is watery and only occasionally contains mucus or blood.

155. The diagnosis of *C. difficile-induced pseudomembranous enterocolitis* is best established by toxin detection. The standard toxin assay is based on neutralization by *Clostridium sordelli* antitoxin. The sensitivity of the test is 95–100%.

156. *Management of pseudomembranous enterocolitis:* (a) Supportive treatment by avoiding antidiarrheal agents and sometimes administration of total parenteral nutrition; (b) vancomycin, 2 g/day orally for 7–14 days; relapse occurs in about 14% of patients, and some patients will have a few episodes of relapse; relapses should be managed with vancomycin as above; (c) cholestyramine, an anion-exchange resin which can bind the C. *difficile* toxin, is recommended for mild to moderate cases; it is less effective than vancomycin but has a lesser rate of relapse; (d) a small minority of patients with pseudomembranous enterocolitis will require diverting ileostomy due to toxic megacolon or refractoriness.

157. Theories to explain the low prevalence of *neoplasia in the small intestine*: (a) rapid transit time; (b) low concentration of bacteria; (c) a developed IgA-mediated immune system; (d) presence of mucosal detoxifying enzymes; (e) reduction of mechanical trauma by liquid chyme; and (f) an alkaline pH.

158. *Leiomyomas of the small intestine* are more common in the jejunum; they tend to bleed and to ulcerate.

159. About 70% of patients with benign *small bowel tumors* have associated benign and malignant tumors in extraintestinal sites.

160. *Osler–Weber–Rendu disease* includes (a) multiple telangiectatic lesions involving the nasopharyngeal, buccal, and gastrointestinal mucosa; (b) repeated hemorrhages from these regions; (c) telangiectatic lesions on the skin, mainly on the palms of the hands and within the nail beds; and (d) familial history of the disorder.

161. *Angiodysplasia*: (a) This arteriovenous malformation occurs predominantly in the cecum and ascending colon; (b) 18% of patients have associated aortic stenosis; (c) a typical angiographic finding is the early opacification of a draining vein during the arterial phase of mesenteric arteriogram; (d) right hemicolectomy is the treatment of choice for lesions that bleed repeatedly.

162. The *"adenoma–carcinoma theory,"* which claims that all or most colonic adenocarcinomas develop within benign adenomas, is still controversial at this writing.

163. The *hyperplastic colonic polyp* is a rearrangement of normal colonic epithelium and need not be removed. *Adenomatous colonic polyps* may grow unrestrainedly and may contain cells that fail to differentiate into mature cell types with many mitoses, so that development into neoplastic lesions is possible only in *adenomatous polyps*.

164. Ninety percent of *colorectal polyps* that are smaller than 3 mm turn out to be *hyperplastic* polyps when examined histologically.

165. In the United States, 50% of the population have at least one *adenomatous polyp* in the large bowel, the majority of which are smaller than 1 cm. In 28% of patients with one colonic adenoma there are multiple adenomatous polyps.

166. *Villous adenomata* tend to be larger in size and of higher malignant potential when compared with *tubular* adenomata.

167. *Adenomatous polyps* located in the distal colon and rectum tend to be larger and are more likely to be malignant.

168. The majority of *colonic adenomas* are asymptomatic. It is assumed that about half of the adenomas bleed but usually in a minor way. Occasional symptoms of lower polypoid lesions include constipation, a sense of fullness in the rectum, and decreased stool caliber. Diarrhea with mucus may be caused by villous adenoma.

169. *Bleeding from colonic polyps* is intermittent in most instances. According to a recent study, 25% of right colonic adenomas and 86% of left colonic adenomas bleed, but the great majority of bleeding episodes result in occult blood in the stool.

170. *Proctosigmoidoscopy* and *testing of stools for occult blood* are the initial screening measures for occult colonic neoplasms.

171. *Guaiac tests* of the stool may lead to false-positive results in up to 50% of asymptomatic patients. The following measures may decrease false-positive results: (a) withdrawal of red meat from the diet for 3 days prior to stool testing; (b) 3 days of high-fiber intake prior to and during stool testing; (c) avoidance of antiinflammatory

drugs and vitamins; (d) testing of two different parts of three separate stools on 3 successive days.

172. When *tests for occult blood* are properly performed, about 30–50%
of asymptomatic patients with positive results will have significant
colorectal lesions detected by diagnostic studies.

173. Both radiologists and colonoscopists may miss *polyps* in the
flexures of the colon, behind the rectal valves, or at the ileocecal
valve.

174. A benign *polyp* found near a cancer in the colon is a harbinger
of a high risk of recurrence. Other risk factors for malignancy in
colonic polyps are the presence of more than one polyp, a high
degree of dysplasia, and a positive family history.

175. *Management of an adenomatous polyp* in the colon: (a) A lesion
less than 0.5 cm in size may be left in place and followed as detailed
below; (b) all polyps on a stalk should be removed at colonoscopy;
(c) large sessile polyps can be removed colonoscopically but the
danger of bleeding and perforation and the likelihood of early
carcinoma make surgical removal preferable; and (d) surgical resection of a colonic segment proximal and distal to an adenomatous
polyp that was removed colonoscopically is indicated when (i) an
undifferentiated carcinoma was found in the polyp; (ii) the carcinoma invades the muscularis mucosa in a sessile polyp; (iii) the
stalk is invaded in a pedunculated polyp; or (iv) cancer is located
at the margin of resection.

176. Most authors agree that simple polypectomy or exfulguration
is adequate therapy for *carcinoma in situ (CIS)* (i.e., when cancerous
cells do not invade the muscularis mucosa) in a pedunculated polyp
unless (a) lymphatics within the polyp contain tumor; (b) the cancer
is highly undifferentiated; or (c) the malignant changes extend to
the neck of the adenoma.

177. The patient who has had a *colonic adenoma* may develop a
second one. Recommended follow-up includes (a) a colonoscopy

or an air-contrast barium enema every 2–3 years after polypectomy of a single benign adenoma; (b) a colonoscopy 6 months after the resection of a polyp that contained CIS or invasive cancer and once a year thereafter; (c) a yearly air-contrast barium enema or colonoscopy in patients with multiple polyps or a strong family history of cancer.

178. *Villous adenoma* (a) comprises 2–14% of all colonic polyps; (b) is more common in the elderly; (c) is most commonly found in the rectosigmoid region, where there is a greater tendency for recurrence and for malignant transformation; (d) may secrete mucus rich in sodium and potassium (hypokalemia is induced only when the lesion is in the anal region and distal reabsorption cannot occur); and (e) occurs as more than one lesion in more than one-third of patients.

179. *Juvenile polyps* are mostly pedunculated, benign, and solitary. They are actually hamartomas that may contain bone tissue, appear at age 1–7 years, and may cause bleeding, diarrhea, or intussusception. Removal of juvenile polyps is suggested because of potential complications, but they disappear with age if not removed.

180. *Inflammatory polyps (pseudopolyps)* reflect a regenerative process surrounded by linear ulcers. They are common in inflammatory bowel disease but may occur in bacterial dysentery, amebic colitis, and schistosomiasis.

181. *Familial polyposis coli (FPC):* (a) It is inherited as an autosomal dominant trait; (b) it is characterized by the development of hundreds to thousands of adenomatous polyps in the large intestine; (c) the development of colon cancer is inevitable if the colon is not removed (most of these patients develop colonic cancer before the age of 40); (d) symptoms are nonspecific and include hematochezia, diarrhea, and abdominal pain; (e) early detection is possible by screening family members of a patient; (f) total colectomy is recommended when the disease is diagnosed; some surgeons recommend the performance of ileorectostomy with flexible sigmoid-oscopy and fulguration of rectal polyps every 6 months; and (g) polyps in the stomach and duodenum may occur.

182. *Gardner's syndrome* is a familial polypsis syndrome with os-teomas, benign skin tumors, thyroid and adrenal tumors, and den-tal abnormalities. It is probably a variant of FPC. Polyps in the stomach and small intestine may occur.

183. *Turcot's syndrome* is another variant of FPC associated with central nervous system tumors (glioblastoma and medulloblas-toma).

184. *Nonfamilial polyposis* of colon, as compared with FPC, is char-acterized by lower frequency of rectal involvement, lower incidence of carcinoma, and higher prevalence in women.

185. *Cronkhite–Canada syndrome* is a *nonfamilial* polyposis of the co-lon, small intestine, and stomach, probably with no increased ten-dency for developing cancer, but with diarrhea, protein-losing en-tropathy, lactase deficiency, and bacterial overgrowth. The polyps are of the inflammatory type, and malabsorption is corrected by antimicrobial agents or TPN. Alopecia, hyperpigmentation, and onychotrophia are associated findings.

186. *Peutz–Jeghers syndrome* is characterized by benign polyposis of stomach, small intestine, and colon with mucocutaneous pigmen-tation. The polyps are hamartomas. The incidence of carcinoma is very low, but obstruction and bleeding may occur.

187. *Carcinoma of the colon and rectum*: (a) This is one of the com-monest cancers of humans—overall it affects 2% of men and 1% of women; (b) the risk for the disease increases significantly at the age of 40 and doubles each decade thereafter; (c) the very high incidence rate and the relatively easy detectability have led some authors to recommend the performance of flexible sigmoidoscopy for every person above 40 or 50 years of age every 3–5 years; and

(d) about 65% of colorectal cancers are within the reach of the standard 60-cm-long flexible sigmoidoscope.

188. Patients with *colorectal cancer* have a 1.5% chance of having a synchronous colorectal cancer, and a 1.5–5% chance of having a metachronous colorectal cancer.

189. The rate of malignant tranformation is 40% for villous adenomas, 5% for tubular adenomas, and 22% for mixed tubulovillous adenomas. Cancer in adenomas is also related to size, 40–50% of adenomas larger than 2 cm showing some focus of cancer as compared with 1% in adenomas of 1 cm or less.

190. In *family cancer syndrome* (a different syndrome from FPC), an autosomal dominant trait for the development of GI and female genital cancers has been shown.

191. The relationship between *family cancer syndrome* and sporadic colon cancer has not been clarified. It has been shown, however, that in first-degree relatives of patients with colorectal cancer, the risk of the disease is three times that in the general population.

192. *Duke's classification* for staging of colonic adenocarcinoma: Stage A: involvement of mucosa and submucosa only; stage B: extension of tumor through all layers of the bowel wall (Astler and Coller modification: B1: muscularis propria is not penentrated, B2: extension through muscularis propria and/or serosa); stage C1: as B1, with lymph node metastases; C2: as B2, with lymph node metastases; and stage D: distant metastatic disease.

193. Commonly cited *5-year survival rates for colorectal carcinoma*: Duke's stage A: 90%; stage B: 70%; stage C: 40%.

194. *Colorectal cancer* is silent during its early development. Early symptoms that may appear: (a) occult blood or gross rectal bleeding (more common when the lesion is on the right side); (b) change in bowel habits or a feeling that the bowel is not really being emptied; (c) crampy, colicky abdominal pain that may represent early ob-

194

struction by the tumor (so may tenesmus and a reduction of stool caliber); and (d) systemic symptoms of malignancy such as weight loss, weakness, malaise, and anorexia.

195. Recommended *screening approach for colorectal cancer*: (a) For average risk groups (patients over 40 years), stool should be examined for occult blood once a year, and a sigmoidoscopy should be done every 3–5 years; a diagnostic work-up using air-contrast barium enema and/or colonoscopy and UGI series should be done in patients with positive findings; (b) for high-risk groups (familial polyposis in the family or family history of colon cancer), air-contrast barium enema and/or colonoscopy should be done at age 20 years, fecal occult blood test once a year, and barium enema and/or colonoscopy every 3 years thereafter; and (c) patients who have had colon cancer or adenoma must be screened radiographically or by colonoscopy for synchronous lesions and every 3–5 years thereafter for the development of new metachromatic lesions.

196. Cure in *colorectal cancer* is expected when 4–5 cm of tumor-free margin are obtained in surgery.

197. In *colorectal cancer* palliative surgery is recommended even in the presence of distant metastases to prevent obstruction, bleeding, or emergency surgery and to relieve cramps and tenesmus in lesions located in the anorectal region.

198. In *colorectal carcinoma* patients with liver metastases have an average survival of 6 months, and patients with solitary liver metastases have an average survival of 16–18 months without treatment and 5-year survival of 20–40% after wedge resection.

199. In one recent study, careful CT scan and ultrasound during the immediate postoperative period after surgery for *colorectal carcinoma* indicated that 25% of patients thought to be cured at surgery had liver metastases (Finlay IG & McCardle CS, Gastroenterology 85:596, 1983).

200. Recurrence after surgery for *colorectal cancer* is common in the suture lines.

201. A recent study on the risk of *colon cancer after cholecystectomy* has indicated (contrary to previous studies) that cholecystectomy reduced the risk of developing this malignancy (Adami HO et al, Gastroenterology 85:859, 1983).

202. *Radiation in colorectal carcinoma* is appropriate (a) for low rectal cancer that is palpable with the finger and appears to be unresectable; (b) preoperatively in patients with epidermiod tumor; (c) postoperatively for pelvic recurrence; and (d) for pain caused by metastases to bone or liver.

203. *Carcinoembryonic antigen (CEA)*: (a) It is disappointing as a screening test; (b) serial determinations are good as an indication for recurrence; and (c) "false" elevations may be encountered in hepatitis, heavy smoking, or transfusion of CEA-positive blood.

204. *Small intestinal malignant tumors* are rare, and the site of highest incidence is the duodenum. Malignant melanoma, breast carcinoma, and lung carcinoma may metastasize to the small intestine and simulate primary small intestinal neoplasia.

205. In *lymphoma of the small intestine*: (a) the lesions are more common in the ileum, where lymph nodes are more prevalent; (b) possible clinical presentations include crampy abdominal pain, bleeding from ulcerations, fever, weight loss, malabsorption, and abdominal mass; perforation occurs in 20–25%; (c) diffuse histiocytic lymphoma is the most common variant; (d) it is difficult to differentiate between primary intestinal lymphoma and involvement of the intestine in generalized lymphoma; (e) management includes resection followed by radiation or chemotherapy; (f) the outlook is poorer than in gastric lymphoma; and (g) there is increased incidence of intestinal lymphoma in celiac disease.

206. *Mediterranean lymphoma*: (a) The duodenum and proximal jejunum are involved; (b) the average age is younger than in intestinal lymphoma (less than 30); (c) it is associated with α-heavy-chain paraproteinemia; (d) it is common among people from the lower socioeconomic classes in the Middle East who have high levels of IgA, which may be due to chronic parasitic infection; and (e) malabsorption with diarrhea and steatorrhea are the prominent symptoms and abdominal pain and clubbing of the fingers are common.

207. The *carcinoid tumor*: (a) It is compatible with long survival even in the presence of metastases; (b) it may originate in the appendix (most common), terminal ileum, rectum, colon, stomach, gallbladder, pancreas, Meckel's diverticle, bronchi, and ovaries; (c) in 20% there is another malignant tumor of the bowel; (d) tumors originating in the small intestine are the most malignant, while those originating in the appendix seldom metastasize; and (e) metastases may cause fibrosis in the retroperitoneum, pleura, and endocardial tissue (valves).

208. *Carcinoid syndrome*: (a) Symptoms induced by serotonin occur only when the hormone is secreted into the systemic circulation (it is inactivated by monoaminoxidase in the liver); (b) principal manifestations include cutaneous flushes, hepatomegaly, diarrhea and abdominal cramps, and endocardial fibrosis with valvular deformity; and (c) other hormones (in addition to serotonin) found in the urine that may induce some of the symptoms are histamine, 5-hydroxytryptophan, bradykinin, prostaglandins, calcitonin, and catecholamines.

209. *Diagnosis of carcinoid syndrome* is made by the finding of >60 mg of 5-hydroxyindoleacetic acid (5-HIAA) in the urine daily. Foods rich in serotonin, such as bananas, pineapples, walnuts, avocados, tomatoes, eggplants, and red plums, should be excluded from the diet. Carcinoid tumor of the stomach and bronchi secretes 5-hydroxytryptophan, which is converted to 5-hydroxytryptamine in the kidneys. The latter is found in elevated levels in the urine.

210. *Management of carcinoid syndrome*: (a) Medical therapy to relieve symptoms includes parachlorophenylalanine to inhibit serotonin synthesis and methysergide maleate to control flushes, asthmatic attacks, and diarrhea (this medication has severe side effects); (b) 5-FU and streptozotocin or adriamycin are a chemotherapeutic option when multiple metastases are present; (c) whole abdominal radiation may improve survival in metastatic tumor; and (d) surgical removal of a large tumor is indicated even in the presence of metastases when the tumor is responsible for mechanical obstruction.

211. *Radiation enteritis and colitis*: (a) Symptoms of acute radiation enteritis include diarrhea, tenesmus, and rectal bleeding; perforation is rare; the clinical and endoscopic presentation is similar to that of acute ulcerative colitis; (b) late intestinal complications of radiation appear from 3 months up to decades after the administration of radiation (usually >4000 rads); the most common presentation is of abdominal cramps with partial small intestinal obstruction; fistulas and abscesses may occur and malabsorption with bacterial overgrowth is not uncommon; and (c) management includes low-fiber diet, antidiarrheal agents, and sedation for the acute stage and steroid enemas and sulfasalazin or surgery to remove strictures in the chronic stage.

212. In the presence of *chronic progressive vascular disease* of the GI tract it is possible for all the intraabdominal viscera to be adequately supplied by only one of the three major mesenteric vessels (the pancreaticoduodenal arcades, the arc of Riolan, and the marginal artery of Drummond) because of anastomotic interconnections.

213. The splenic flexure and the junction of the superior and middle portions of the rectum are vulnerable to *ischemia*. In these regions of the colon, branches of the inferior mesenteric artery anastomose with branches of the superior mesenteric artery (splenic flexure) and hypogastric arteries (rectum).

214. *Digitalis glycosides* have been shown to cause vasoconstriction of blood vessels supplying the GI tract.

215. *Acute occlusion* of one of the three major blood vessels of the GI tract may result in ischemic necrosis. It is more common in the superior mesenteric artery, which has a relatively large caliber, and it takes off from the aorta rather obliquely. Emboli occur less commonly in the celiac axis, as it originates from the aorta at almost a right angle, or in the inferior mesenteric artery, due to its relatively small caliber.

216. *Clinical features of intestinal angina*: (a) severe postprandial colicky abdominal pain occurring 20–30 min after a large meal (between meals the patient is pain free; the pain leads to a fear of eating); (b) weight loss (malabsorption is extremely uncommon); and (c) the fact that the history is the main clue to the diagnosis; other diagnostic studies are of little help, even including angiography, which shows the vessel diameter but does not measure blood flow.

217. In *extensive bowel infarction* severe abdominal pain and distention are the prominent clinical features. Vomiting is common, and hematemesis or rectal bleeding may occur. Early in the course, there is no significant objective abdominal finding, and the earliest sign may be hyperperistalsis. Later in the course, distention, tenderness, and other signs of peritonitis appear. An elderly patient with congestive heart failure and/or atrial fibrillation is the "typical" candidate to develop the syndrome. Fever (up to 39–40°C) and leukocytosis are common.

218. *Diagnostic approach to suspected bowel infarction*: (a) Plain abdominal film may show complete absence of air in the small bowel initially and generalized distention later; thickened edematous wall may be seen in patients with ischemic colitis; gas in the portal vein is evidence of a leak of bacteria from the infarcted gut; (b) if plain abdominal films are equivocal, an early barium enema is indicated;

spasm, narrowing, irritability, and thumbprints representing mucosal edema are typical; later, ulceration and fibrosis may appear; (c) the need for an angiographic study is not absolute; in almost 75% of the patients there will be no demonstrable blockage even if a segment of necrotic bowel is found at surgery; and (d) colonoscopy is not contraindicated, and it may lend support to the diagnosis; findings include swollen mucosal folds and a dusky mucosa containing multiple ulcerations similar to those seen in Crohn's disease.

219. *Bowel infarction* is an indication for immediate surgery (while the bowel is still viable). Patients should be prepared with restoation of intravascular volume and coverage with antimicrobial agents. Congestive heart failure should be treated as efficiently as possible. The place of intraarterial infusion of vasodilators is uncertain, but most authors recommend their use. At surgery the necrotic bowel should be resected and, if the patient is sufficiently stable, an attempt should be made to revascularize the remaining viable bowel by bypass graft, embolectomy, or endarterectomy. Methods to define intraoperatively the limits of viable bowel include visual assessment of color and peristalsis, palpation of mesenteric pulses, electromyography, Doppler ultrasonography, injection of radioactive microspheres, and fluorescein angiography. A "second-look" operation is frequently needed 12–36 hr after the initial surgery.

220. *Celiac axis compression syndrome* characterized by recurrent abdominal pain associated with narrowing of the celiac axis (compressed by the median arcuate ligament of the diaphragm) is a controversial entity. If the syndrome does exist it is an exception to the rule that at least two major visceral arteries must be narrowed before symptoms occur.

221. *Mesenteric venous thrombosis*: (a) It is associated with disorders predisposing to stasis (congestive heart failure, portal hypertension, abdominal neoplasm), intraabdominal infections, and hypercoagulable states; (b) in 98% of patients the thrombotic process is in the superior mesenteric vein; (c) clinical features are similar to those seen in arterial infarction; (d) surgery to remove necrotic bowel is indicated.

222. *Aortoenteric fistula* occurs in 1–2% of patients after resection of an abdominal aortic aneurysm and its replacement by graft. The fistula usually forms between the graft and the third portion of the duodenum. Recurrent episodes of minor bleeding commonly precede massive, difficult-to-control bleeding.

4
Inflammatory Bowel Disease

1. *Inflammatory bowel disease (IBD)* is a spectrum of disorders including regional enteritis, ulcerative colitis, and Crohn's colitis. It is difficult to distinguish Crohn's colitis from ulcerative colitis on clinical, radiological, and even pathological grounds.

2. *Regional enteritis* occurs more frequently in Ashkenazi Jews. The average age of onset is about 27 years, but the disease may first appear in childhood or in old age. Male/female ratio is 1:1–1.6.

3. *Pathological findings in regional enteritis* include (a) an inflammatory process extending through all layers of the bowel wall; (b) thickening of the bowel wall with narrowing of the lumen, thickening of the mesentery, enlarged mesenteric lymph nodes and adhesions between adjacent loops of the bowel; and (c) hyperplasia of perilymphatic histiocytes, a diffuse granulomatous infiltration, noncaseating granulomata in the submucosa and lamina propria, and small aphthous ulcerations overlying Peyer's patches.

4. *Granulomas in Crohn's disease* (a) when absent do not exclude the diagnosis; (b) occasionally (10% of the granulomas) contain Shau-

mann bodies (as in foreign body granulomas); (c) may occur in the liver and other organs in the vicinity of the diseased bowel; (d) are more common in the colon and anus than in the small bowel; (e) decrease in number with duration of symptoms; and (f) may be associated with better prognosis and less chance of recurrence (controversial).

5. In *Crohn's disease*, more than two-thirds of patients have small intestine involvement and two-thirds show colon involvement (ileocolitis), but in only 10–25% of cases is the colon alone involved (Crohn's colitis).

6. *Diarrhea in Crohn's disease* is the most common clinical feature (90% of patients). It is more severe when the colon is involved than when the disease is limited to the small bowel. Frequent diarrhea with urgency, tenesmus, and incontinence is also indicative of colonic involvement.

7. *Abdominal pain* is the second most common symptom in *Crohn's disease* (76%). It is usually a chronic steady ache in the right lower quadrant and becomes colicky when small intestinal obstruction is superimposed.

8. *Fever* is the third most common symptom in Crohn's disease (40%). It is usually low-grade and temperatures above 39°C (102°F) indicate an intraabdominal abscess or fistula formation. Fever may be the only manifestation of the disease for weeks or months.

9. *Bleeding in Crohn's disease* occurs in about 50% of patients sometime during the course of the disease. It is uncommon in the initial stage, when the process is mainly submucosal, and becomes more common when mucosal fissures and ulcerations occur. Massive bleeding is uncommon.

10. *Fistulas in Crohn's disease* are common and lead to a variety of other complications. Perianal and perirectal fistulas and fissures are particularly common. Enteroenteric and enterocutaneous fistulas occur more frequently in patients with ileocolonic involve-

5 _____

ment than among those with Crohn's disease involving only the small intestine or the colon. Fistulas may lead to nutritional problems if extensive segments of the small intestine are bypassed or to bacterial overgrowth due to stasis. Enterovesical fistulas are infrequent and lead to pneumaturia and persistent urinary tract infection (UTI).

11. *Free perforation in Crohn's disease* is unusual, but walled-off abscesses are common.

12. *Extraintestinal complications of Crohn's disease* are more common when there is colonic and/or perianal involvement. They include arthritis (migratory of large joints or spondylitis–sacroileitis), iritis, episcleritis, erythema nodosum, pyoderma gangrenosum, and aphthous stomatitis. Nephrolithiasis (from hyperoxaluria) occurs in 25–35% of cases.

13. *Hepatobiliary complications of Crohn's disease* include (a) pericholangitis; (b) diffuse or focal granulomatous inflammation; (c) sclerosing cholangitis; (d) cholangiocarcinoma (rare); and (e) cholelithiasis in about 30% of patients.

14. The most useful *diagnostic aid when Crohn's disease is suspected* is barium enema. Every effort should be made to get the barium to pass from the cecum into the small bowel. Involvement of terminal ileum and proximal colon is suggestive of Crohn's disease.

15. In patients acutely ill with *Crohn's disease,* barium enema is not recommended, but the danger of perforation is less than in ulcerative colitis.

16. The *Crohn's Disease Actitivy Index* suggested by the National Cooperative Study Group during the late 1970s (Best WR et al, Gastroenterology 70:439, 1976) has not proved clinically useful. Acute-phase reactants, such as *sedimentation rate, C-reactive protein,* and *serum orosomucoid* have been found to correlate best with clinical assessment of the patient.

17. *Bacterial overgrowth (BOG)* may occur in up to two-thirds of patients with Crohn's disease. *Escherichia coli* is the predominant bacterium. BOG is most likely to occur when there is an element of stasis or obstruction.

18. Possible *radiological findings in Crohn's disease* include (a) linear ulcers; (b) internal fistulas; (c) cobblestoning; (d) stenosis (string sign); and (e) skip lesions. Findings are most common in the terminal ileum, cecum, and ascending colon and in regions of previous anastomoses.

19. In *Crohn's disease* there is poor correlation between the radiographic appearance and the clinical state. There is no indication for repeated X-ray examinations to evaluate progress or response to therapy.

20. Duodenal abnormalities may be seen radiographically in up to 22% of patients with *Crohn's disease*. Duodenal ulcer disease, particularly postbulbar ulcer, must be differentiated from Crohn's disease.

21. Both ultrasonography and CT scanning are useful in evaluating right lower quadrant masses in *Crohn's disease* to determine whether an abscess is present.

22. General guidelines for the *management of Crohn's disease* are as follows: (a) administration of no agents to an asymptomatic patient (when terminal ileitis has been discovered on X-ray examination or during surgery for appendicitis); (b) bed rest and antidiarrheal agents for active disease with diarrhea; (c) intravenous fluids in acute attacks; (d) N-G tube in obstruction; (e) IV antimicrobial agents when an abscess is suspected; and (f) emotional support.

23. The role of *diet* in the management of symptomatic *Crohn's disease* is controversial. Some authorities recommend a low-residue diet when diarrhea is the main clinical symptom; others claim there is no evidence that what the patient eats affects the symptoms or the course. Low-residue diet has been recommended by all for patients with narrowing of the gut lumen and a propensity for obstructive episodes. Lactose intolerance should be considered, since it is not uncommon in its acquired form in patients with Crohn's disease.

24. *Drug treatment in active Crohn's disease*: (a) should be given to patients whose symptoms are unrelieved by bed rest and supportive treatment; (b) *sulfasalazine*, 1.0 g/15 kg: most effective in previously untreated patients, in unoperated patients, and in those with colonic involvement, in treating symptomatic disease, but is no more effective than placebo in preventing recurrences; patients treated with sufasalazine should regularly receive folic acid supplementation; (c) *prednisone*, 0.25–0.75 mg/kg: more effective early during the course of the disease and in patients previously untreated with drugs; less effective in disease limited to the colon; in severely sick patients, hydrocortisone, 300 mg/day, IV; whenever steroid treatment is commenced, the dose should be reduced as soon as symptomatic relief occurs to that amount which will control symptoms (if the patient becomes asymptomatic on a small dose, a trial to omit steroids should be conducted); (d) *sulfasalazine + prednisone*: appears to be no more effective than prednisone alone in suppressing the acute attack or in preventing recurrence; (e) *azathioprine* or *6-mercaptopurine*: shown to have a steroid-"sparing" effect; should be considered a therapeutic option in patients with persistent severe disease that has not responded to treatment with sulfasalazine, corticosteroids, and resective therapy or in those patients in whom reduction in steroid dosage is badly needed; (f) *5-aminosalicylic acid (5-ASA)*, one of the two metabolites of sulfasalazine, is probably the active constituent of sulfasalazine; beneficial effects of this agent over sulfasalazine in the treatment of Crohn's disease have yet to be determined; and (g) *metronidazole*, 1–1.5 g/day: shown, in a limited number of studies, to be effective in healing perianal involvement in Crohn's disease, but relapses were common after reduction of the dose or cessation of therapy.

25. *Nutritional considerations in Crohn's disease*: (a) low-residue diet is recommended when diarrhea is the dominating symptom; (b) specific replacement of vitamin D, calcium, folic acid, iron, and other nutrients is indicated whenever there is clinical or laboratory evidence of deficiency; (c) after ileal resection, supplementation of vitamin B_{12} and substitution of medium-chain triglycerides for long-chain triglycerides in the diet may be necessary; (d) elimination of milk or milk products from the diet is recommended in patients with proven lactose intolerance; (e) elemental diets and TPN have proved ineffective in the long-term management of Crohn's disease; transient improvement and healing of fistulas have been observed in patients receiving TPN, but high relapse rates (up to 80% within 3 months) have occurred after discontinuation of treatment; aggressive nutritional therapy is justified to prevent or reverse growth retardation and delayed sexual maturation in children and adolescents with severe disease.

26. A recent study on the *natural history of Crohn's disease* has shown that 41% of patients improved spontaneously within 3–4 months of follow-up (Meyers S & Janowitz HD, Gastroenterology 87:1189, 1984).

27. *Surgery in Crohn's disease* involves several considerations: (a) it should be considered only in patients refractory to medical therapy for alleviation of intractable symptoms or for therapy of complications such as intestinal obstruction, persistent external fistula, or anal disease; (b) in about 50–70% of patients with Crohn's disease, complications will develop at one time or another requiring surgery, and recurrent disease will occur sometime after surgery in the vast majority of cases; about 25% of patients operated on will require another resection; (c) when acute Crohn's disease is discovered during laparotomy for suspected appendicitis, resection should not be performed because most cases of acute enteritis are self-limited; the appendix may be removed at the time of laparotomy if there is no inflammatory involvement of the base of the appendix or of the cecum; (d) most surgeons resect only segments with gross disease, preserving as much small intestine as possible and paying no attention to microscopic evidence of disease; (e) bypass operations are not recommended because of higher risk of recurrence and a slightly increased risk of cancer in the bypassed loop; resection is preferable; (f) not all fistulas require surgery—fistulas may disappear spontaneously (however, rectal or vaginal fistulas or marked anal disease are very disabling and necessitate an operation; fistulous tracts to the bladder should be repaired without delay); (g) ileorectostomy is the preferred operation for patients with Crohn's colitis or ileocolitis in whom the rectum is normal, although the rate of rectal recurrence is high (recent studies indicate that ileorectostomy may be considered even when the rectum is mildly or moderately involved—in one study, 20% of patients required an ileostomy within 5 years of initial operation; and (h) improved surgical techniques nowadays enable the removal of rectal mucosa with preservation of the rectal musculature; the ileum is then joined to the anus and conventional rectal continence is maintained.

28. Expected complications after *resection of the terminal ileum* include (a) B_{12} deficiency (1000 µg of B_{12} IM should be given every 3 months); (b) nephrolithiasis with calcium oxalate stones; (c) cholelithiasis due to reduced absorption of bile salts; and (d) steatorrhea and/or cholerrheic diarrhea.

29. In *Crohn's disease,* involvement of parts of the GI tract other than the ileum and colon (jejunum, duodenum, stomach, esophagus, oral mucosa) causes symptoms that are entirely nonspecific. Weight loss, nausea, vomiting, and peptic-ulcer-like symptoms may occur.

30. *Carcinoma in Crohn's disease*: The association of Crohn's disease and small bowel adenocarcinoma is a rare but well-documented condition. It occurs in no more than 0.3% of patients with Crohn's disease, usually after many years have elapsed since the diagnosis of regional enteritis. It occurs in a younger age group compared with small bowel carcinoma unassociated with Crohn's disease. It is more frequently located in the terminal ileum and tends to be multifocal. Prognosis is extremely poor, and there are no 5-year survivors. Bypassed segments of the intestine tend to develop the malignant process—one of the arguments against the performance of bypass surgery in Crohn's disease. Carcinoma of the colon occurs in Crohn's colitis, but precise figures for incidence are not yet clear.

31. *Crohn's colitis* as opposed to ulcerative colitis is characterized by (a) skip lesions; (b) granulomas found in up to 75% of biopsies; (c) sparing of the rectum (common); (d) perianal disease (common); (e) massive bleeding (more common, although the number of bleeding episodes is larger in ulcerative colitis); and (f) less toxicity (perforations and toxic megacolon are uncommon).

32. The principles underlining the *management of Crohn's colitis* are similar to those for the management of regional enteritis, but steroids are less effective and there is a strong clinical impression that they predispose to the development of anal and abdominal fistulas and may even prevent their healing. Sulfasalazine is more effective in Crohn's colitis than in regional enteritis, and steroids should be reserved for moderate to severe cases when other measures fail to return the patient to good health. Some authorities recommend the use of 6-mercaptopurine or azathioprine in refractory patients with extensive small intestinal and colonic involvement. Metronidazole should be tried in refractory perianal disease.

33. The *surgical approach to Crohn's colitis* is the same as that for regional enteritis: The patient should be treated medically as long as possible and by the minimal operation when medical measures have failed. Chances of recurrence of Crohn's colitis after surgery are very high, running between 60% and 100% according to different investigators. When surgery is unavoidable, colectomy with ileostomy is the most common procedure. Recent reports indicate, however, that ileorectostomy, even when the rectum is mildly or moderately involved, has led to satisfactory results, with about 20% of patients requiring removal of the ileostomy within 5 years. Newer techniques to preserve the anal site of defecation include removal of the rectal mucosa, preserving the rectal musculature and then joining the ileum to the anus or creating an ileal reservoir much like the Kock ileostomy.

34. The *Copenhagen Crohn's Study* published in February 1985 shows that only a small minority of patients are continuously symptomatic (with or without therapy). A mean follow-up period of 55 years indicated that most led normal active lives and that mortality is similar to that in the general population (Binder V et al, Gut 26:146, 1985).

35. *Epidemiology of ulcerative colitis:* It (a) is more common in Jews (two- to fourfold); (b) is more common in whites than in blacks (fourfold); (c) appears to be a disease of urban life; (d) shows a family history of the disease in about 20% of patients; and (e) shows an increased frequency of HLA-11 and HLA-7 and a reduced frequency of HLA-3.

36. *Ulcerative colitis* is limited to the mucosa, with occasional involvement of the submucosa. The serosa and regional lymph nodes are never involved.

37. *Histological changes in ulcerative colitis* include (a) reduced number of goblet cells; (b) microabscesses; (c) microscopic ulcerations formed by the coalescence of adjacent microabscesses; and (d) increased number of paneth cells (limited to the area above the rectosigmoid).

38. *Backwash ileitis* is the involvement of the distal small bowel in ulcerative colitis. It occurs in about one-third of patients. It is of no clinical or prognostic significance.

39. The *clinical course of ulcerative colitis* is characterized by intermittent attacks of symptoms with complete symptomatic remissions between attacks in 60–75% of patients, by continuous symptoms without any remission in 5–15%, and by one attack with no subsequent symptoms for many years in 4–10%.

40. *Symptoms of ulcerative colitis* include (a) diarrhea; (b) abdominal cramps; (c) anorexia and weight loss; (d) fever; and (e) weakness, lassitude, and general feeling of illness.

41. In *clinically mild ulcerative colitis*, (a) disease is frequently limited to the rectosigmoid (80%) but may affect the whole colon; (b) mild diarrhea (3–4 times a day) is common; (c) patients may note blood in the stool; (d) severe abdominal cramps, fever, and weight loss are uncommon, and general health is unimpaired; (e) mortality is near zero and prognosis is not significantly different from that in the general population; and (f) carcinoma is seven times less common than in the severe form of the disease.

42. In *clinically moderate ulcerative colitis* (a), there are more than five bowel movements per day; (b) low-grade fever and abdominal cramps are common; (c) extracolonic symptoms such as low backache, arthritis, or uveitis are more common than in the mild form; (d) the most dramatic symptomatic response to steroid therapy is observed in this group, but long-term prognosis remains poor; and (e) the risk of ultimate development of cancer is appreciable.

43. *Severe or fulminant ulcerative colitis* (a) is the least common form, affecting about 15% of patients; (b) is manifested by sudden onset of symptoms (common); (c) is characterized by profuse bloody diarrhea, severe abdominal cramps, fever, tenesmus, anorexia, fatigue, and dehydration; (d) may include constipation when the disease is limited to the rectosigmoid; (e) is often refractory to medical treatment and mortality rate is high (27% according to one report); and (f) displays extracolonic manifestations more commonly than in other forms and includes (in addition to the above), aphthous stomatitis, erythema nodosum, and pyoderma gangrenosum.

44. *Findings on sigmoidoscopy in ulcerative colitis* are as follows: (a) the mucosa is less transluscent than normal due to submucosal inflammation and edema, and the normal vascular pattern disappears; (b) the mucosal surface is irregular in height and depth and appears granular when examined tangentially; (c) the mucosa is friable, i.e., bleeds easily from punctate bleeding sites when gently massaged; (d) spontaneous bleeding may occur in more advanced disease; (e) discrete ulcerations are uncommon in the rectosigmoid; and (f) pseudopolyps can be seen in severe forms of the disease.

45. In *ulcerative colitis,* the severity of the clinical picture correlates poorly with the endoscopic appearance.

46. The endoscopic differentiation between *ulcerative colitis* and acute *amebic colitis* is difficult. Treatment for ulcerative colitis should not be started before excluding amebic colitis by culturing stool for amebae.

47. *Colonoscopy* should not be performed in the setting of *acute severe ulcerative colitis* because of the risk of perforation. However, perforations have been reported rarely when the flexible sigmoidoscope was used.

48. *Barium enema* is less sensitive than colonoscopy in diagnosing *ulcerative colitis,* but the double-contrast technique increases sensitivity, and a diffusely granular appearance comparable to that seen on colonoscopy can be recognized quite clearly during the course of the disease. Barium enema should not be performed during the severely active phase of ulcerative colitis. Patients receiving barium enema during quiescent periods of the disease should not have vigorous preparation with purgatives or enemas but mild saline cathartics such as magnesium citrate and 48-hr liquid diet.

49. Barium enema or sigmoidoscopy are not recommended for follow-up of patients with *ulcerative colitis* because of the small correlation between prognosis and radiographic or endoscopic appearance and because of the risk of precipitating an exacerbation or perforation. Barium enema study or endoscopy are indicated when the illness recurs after a period of remission or when symptoms dramatically intensify or to exclude the appearance of carcinoma in long-standing disease.

50. In correcting dehydration caused by diarrhea of *ulcerative colitis,* colonic losses of sodium and potassium (in addition to fluid loss) should be accounted for.

51. The use of opiates for symptomatic relief of diarrhea in moderate or severe *ulcerative colitis* is contraindicated, as they may contribute to the development of *toxic megacolon.*

52. *Steroids in the management of ulcerative colitis:* (a) corticosteroid therapy may induce remission or improvement in the acute attack, but the long-term benefits have yet to be assessed; (b) at acceptable dose, steroids do not prevent relapse; (c) in patients with mild disease, especially when limited to the distal colon, rectal instillation of steroids induces or maintains remission in most cases; 100–200 mg hydrocortisone in 120–150 ml saline can be administered rectally with change of position every 20 min after instillation to permit maximal topical coverage; (d) steroid foam preparations reach only as far as the sigmoid colon, while the regular steroid enema fluid may be carried more proximally; (e) rectally administered steroids probably exert their effect both locally and through systemic absorption; (f) in severe ulcerative colitis, 300 mg hydrocortisone or 100 mg prednisolone should be administered IV daily for 10–14 days; if response is observed, this should be followed by oral prednisolone with gradual tapering; (g) steroids should not be given during complete remission, but if high-dose steroids do not lead to complete remission, long-term, low-dose steroids should be considered; if the patient requires more than 15 mg oral prednisone daily for months to control the colitis and/or extracolonic complications, elective colectomy should be considered.

53. *Sulfasalazine in the management of ulcerative colitis*: (a) it is useful for prevention of relapse; (b) its action in healing colitis is less than the action of oral steroids and occurs at a slower rate and should not be relied on solely as a treatment for severe disease; (c) for prevention of relapses sulfasalazine should be given at a dose of 2 g/day for at least 1 year; (d) sulfasalazine has many side effects, e.g., nausea, vomiting, headache, male infertility, hemolytic anemia (in G6PD deficiency), and allergic reactions; (e) rectal administration of sulfasalazine has proved as effective as oral therapy and is associated with fewer side effects; and (f) 5-ASA appears to be the active constituent of sulfasalazine; several preparations have recently been described that release 5-ASA in the lower intestine. Their expected benefit and fewer side effects compared with sulfasalazine have yet to be determined.

54. *Immunosuppressive agents in the management of ulcerative colitis*: Most authors agree that azathioprine, or other immunosuppressive agents, have little to offer in most cases of ulcerative colitis and that the use of potentially dangerous drugs in patients who can be cured by surgery is unjustified.

55. *Medical therapy of ulcerative colitis* is designed to achieve three goals: (a) to terminate the acute attack; (b) to prevent recurrences; and (c) to allow a timely decision on surgical approach when medical therapy is exhausted or life-threatening complications occur during medical treatment.

56. In *ulcerative colitis*, the first attack carries a mortality of 4–6%. The severity of the clinical illness is the most predictive factor of mortality. The extent of colonic involvement roughly correlates with clinical severity. Mortality is highest among those below the age of 20 and those over 60 years. The initial attack is mild in 60% of patients, moderate in 25%, and severe in 15%.

57. *Pregnancy and ulcerative colitis*: (a) the disease has no effect on female fertility; (b) the incidence of congenital abnormalities and spontaneous abortions is equivalent to that noted in the general population; (c) the relapse rate of ulcerative colitis in remission during pregnancy is not significantly different from the relapse rate of the disease in nonpregnant patients within the same period of time, but most relapses occur during the first trimester or during the postpartum period; (d) when ulcerative colitis is active at the time of conception, it will remain active in about 50% of women, 20% may experience improvement, and the rest are unaffected by the pregnancy; and (e) management of the disease during pregnancy does not differ from that of the nonpregnant patient with . ulcerative colitis; therapeutic abortion is unwarranted, as it will not improve even a severe attack.

58. *Indications for definitive surgery in ulcerative colitis*: (a) a patient acutely ill with ulcerative colitis who shows no signs of response after 5–10 days on IV steroid therapy; (c) free perforation; (d) rectovaginal fistula; (e) chronic relapsing disease when relief requires restriction of the patient's daily activities for a significant period; (f) chronic (about 1 year) downhill course despite optimal medical therapy; and (g) suspected or proved colonic cancer (note: in contrast to surgery in Crohn's disease, removal of the colon in ulcerative colitis is curative in most instances).

59. *Type of surgery for ulcerative colitis*: (a) it is generally agreed that the standard surgical procedure is proctocolectomy with an ileostomy when the rectum is involved in the disease because of high incidence of diarrhea, bleeding, perirectal inflammation, and carcinoma if the involved rectum is left behind; (b) ileorectostomy when the rectum is not involved has gained some popularity lately and is sometimes done with extirpation of the rectal mucosa; it is too early to assess the long-term results in terms of recurrence of the disease in the stump or the development of carcinoma; (c) in

57 ───

Park's procedure, an ileal reservoir, similar to that constructed by Kock for ileostomy, is fashioned just before the anal sphincter and patients may have perianal control; this type of surgery is still experimental; (d) when proctocolectomy is done, some surgeons construct Kock's continent ileostomy as an alternative to the conventional stoma; results are better than in Crohn's disease, where ileitis in the reservoir loop is common, but even in ulcerative colitis 25% of patients will require revision of the nipple stoma.

60. In elective colectomy for *ulcerative colitis*, postoperative mortality is about 3%. It is 10–15% in patients undergoing emergency surgery for acute severe disease and around 50% in critically ill patients being operated for colonic perforation.

61. *Common complications after proctocolectomy for ulcerative colitis*: (a) impotence occurs in 10% of operated patients and is almost always temporary (average duration 1 year); (b) prolonged perineal drainage and slow healing; (c) dyspareunia and infertility occur in female patients (uncommon complications); and (d) in the vast majority of patients, no major complications develop and excellent general health can be expected.

62. *The role of hyperalimentation in the treatment of ulcerative colitis*: as in Crohn's disease, does not abort the course of disease. It is recommended in malnourished anorectic patients, especially in preparation for surgery.

63. In *children with ulcerative colitis*, the rectum is almost always involved. Long-term prognosis is poor, as cancer develops within 14 years in about 10% of patients. Life expectancy is also shortened by nonmalignant complications. In one large study, mortality was 20% after 10 years, and about 40% of the children whose ulcerative colitis started in childhood did not survive 20 years after development of the disease. For all these reasons, total colectomy should be considered early in the course of ulcerative colitis in children.

64. *Minor local complications of ulcerative colitis* include (a) hemorrhoids (20%); (b) pseudopolyps (15%); (c) anal fissures (12%); (d) anal fistulas (5%); (e) perianal abscesses (5%); (f) rectal prolapse (2%); and (g) rectovaginal fistulas (2.5%).

65. *Major local complications of ulcerative colitis* include the following: (a) *Toxic megacolon*: this is an acute dilatation of all or part of the colon to a diameter greater than 6 cm (measured in midtransverse colon) associated with systemic toxicity; it occurs in about 1.5% of patients with ulcerative colitis and in about 10% of patients hospitalized for this disease, more commonly among the young. Perforation is a common complication of toxic megacolon. Toxic megacolon should be managed initially by IV steroids, antimicrobial agents, N-G tube, moving the patient from one position to another to move the gas along the colon, albumin, and blood as necessary. Opiates should be stopped. A thorough physical examination of the abdomen and plain abdominal radiography should be done daily in a search for signs of colonic perforation. Total colectomy should be performed if there has not been substantial deflation of the bowel within 48–72 hr. Mortality from toxic megacolon is around 15%.

(b) *Colonic perforation* without toxic megacolon: This occurs in 3% of patients with ulcerative colitis. Corticosteroids may mask symptoms and signs of perforation. Surgery is indicated immediately when perforation is diagnosed or suspected; even then, operative mortality is around 50%. Continued medical treatment when perforation occurs results in approximately 80% mortality. Colonic perforation accounts for about one-third of deaths directly related to colitis.

(c) *Cancer of the colon*: This malignancy is much more common in patients with ulcerative colitis as compared with the general population. It has been claimed that 5–10% of patients with ulcerative colitis develop colonic cancer sometime during the course of the disease and that 5–8% will develop the malignant complication after 15 years from onset, 12% after 20 years, and 25% after 25 years. However, a few recent papers claim that the incidence of colonic cancer in ulcerative colitis is much lower. In the Copenhagen Ulcerative Colitis Study, 7 of 783 patients developed colonic cancer after an average follow-up of 6.7 years (Hendriksen et al, Gut 26:158, 1985). Another study on 959 patients indicated no cases of cancer after 10 years from onset, 5% after 20 years, 15% after 30 years, and 20% after 35 years. Cancer in ulcerative colitis occurs in a younger age than the same process in the general population, is more common in extensive involvement of the colon, and quiescence of the colitis is no guarantee that carcinoma will not develop. Dysplasia of colonic epithelium (increased nuclear size, crowding of nuclei, loss of nuclear polarity, and depletion of mucin) is considered a marker of colonic cancer in ulcerative colitis, although there is a false-negative rate of 12% and a false-positive rate of 13%. Dysplasia is more sensitive for colonic carcinoma when it is present in the colon than in the rectum. Different investigators recommend different surveillance programs for early detection of colonic cancer in patients with ulcerative colitis, but all agree that colonoscopy with biopsies taken at 10-cm intervals along the colon should be performed beginning 10 years after onset of colitis. If dysplasia is found colonoscopy should be repeated annually. Total colectomy is suggested for patients with severe dysplastic changes or when a polypoid mass that is not a pseudopolyp is found at colonoscopy. Overall 5-year survival is the same (33%) for colonic carcinoma diagnosed in an otherwise normal colon or in a colon with ulcerative colitis, although one would expect survival to be better in a carefully monitored colon.

(d) *Colonic stricture*: This problem occurs in 7–11% of patients with ulcerative colitis as a result of muscular hypertrophy. It is commonly asymptomatic and is discovered initially during routine barium enema, but distinction from cancer is difficult and surgery is indicated.

(e) *Massive hemorrhage*: This is uncommon and occurs in 4% of cases, mostly with severe colitis. The bleeding usually stops spontaneously, but occasionally colectomy is required.

66. *Extracolonic complications of ulcerative colitis* include (a) arthritis: affects about 15–20% of patients; may be monoarticular, but may also involve many joints at once, most frequently the large joints; joint symptoms wax and wane with activity of the intestinal disease, usually respond to steroids, and, if refractory, may be relieved by colectomy; (b) ankylosing spondylitis: 10–20 times as frequent in ulcerative colitis as in the general population; (c) clinically significant aortic stenosis is observed in 2–6% of patients, (d) iritis, episcleritis, erythema nodosum, and pyoderma gangrenosum: occur in a small minority of patients, usually during exacerbation of the colitis; (e) liver disease: common, but only 1–2% of patients will have overt liver disease, mainly when the colitis is extensive; types of liver disease include fatty infiltration, pericholangitis, chronic active hepatitis (rare), sclerosing cholangitis, portal fibrosis and cirrhosis, and amyloidosis; carcinoma of bile ducts complicates ulcerative colitis in 0.5% of cases; colectomy does not affect liver disease in ulcerative colitis; (f) pyelonephritis and nephrolithiasis with calcium oxalate or uric acid stones; and (g) iron deficiency anemia (bleeding) and Coombs-positive hemolytic anemia; as well as thromboembolic phenomena (uncommon).

67. *Hyposplenism* has been commonly reported in inflammatory bowel disease. This complication occurs in Crohn's disease only when the colon is involved; it is associated with severity of the disease.

5
The Pancreas

1. The pancreas is 12–15 cm long and weighs 70–110 g in the adult.

2. *Blood supply to the pancreas* is through (a) the anterior and posterior superior pancreaticoduodenal arteries, which arise as branches of the gastroduodenal artery, a branch of the celiac artery; (b) the anterior and posterior inferior pancreaticoduodenal arteries, which are branches of the superior mesenteric artery; and (c) the splenic artery, which gives rise to the dorsal pancreatic artery, the pancreatica magna, the cauda pancreatis, and numerous small branches.

3. *Venous drainage of the pancreas* is into the portal venous system through the pancreatic veins, which join the splenic vein, and through the pancreaticoduodenal veins, which empty either into the splenic vein or directly into the portal vein.

4. The *pancreas secretes 500–2000 ml* of an alkaline fluid (pH 8) daily but has the capacity to secrete twice this amount. The fluid is composed of water, electrolytes, and bicarbonate (contributed mainly by the ductular cells) and of enzymes that help digest fat, protein, and carbohydrates (e.g., amylase, trypsin, and lipase secreted by the acinar cells).

4

5. The human pancreas contains about one million *islets of Langerhans*.

6. In the *exocrine pancreas*, each cell type secretes several different digestive enzymes, while in the *endocrine pancreas* each cell type secretes a single hormone. *Beta cells*, 75–80% of the islets, secrete insulin; *alpha cells*, 10–20% of the cell mass, secrete glucagon; and *delta cells*, 5% of the islets, secrete somatostatin.

7. Usually the *major pancreatic duct (Wirsung)* enters the duodenum at the ampulla of Vater alongside the common bile duct, and both ducts are encased in the sphincter of Oddi. In 30–40% of individuals, both ducts form a common channel before terminating.

8. The major secretion of the pancreas is under duodenal and intestinal control, through the action of *secretin* and *CCK*. There is also a nervous phase (central or vagal) that is responsible for secretion of fluid rich in enzymes and low in bicarbonate. Secretion of secretin from the duodenal mucosa is evoked by the presence of acid in the duodenal lumen; this hormone stimulates the outflow of pancreatic secretion high in bicarbonate and relatively low in enzymes. Amino acids and fatty acids stimulate duodenal release of CCK, which stimulates pancreatic secretion (rich in enzymes, low in water and bicarbonate).

9. The *pancreas has a remarkable reserve capacity*, and fat or protein are not lost in the stool until lipase and trypsin output is reduced to 10% of normal. Moreover, alternative pathways of digestion do exist, as up to 40% of dietary fat and protein may be assimilated in the absence of pancreatic enzymes.

10. *Cystic fibrosis* is characterized as follows: (a) it is the most common lethal genetic defect in Caucasians; (b) 80% of patients live beyond the age of 20, some of whom are not diagnosed until the second or third decade of life; (c) in 99% of patients the "sweat test" is positive, i.e., sweat contains more than 77 mEq/liter Cl^-

and more than 74 mEq/liter Na $^+$; (d) rectal prolapse and meconium ileus are common in children, and nasal polyps are common in adults with this disease; (e) liver and biliary tract manifestations include *fatty liver, focal biliary cirrhosis, gallstones, small gallbladder,* and *cholecystitis*; (f) fat and protein maldigestion and fecal loss are the primary manifestations of pancreatic involvement; on duodenal aspiration, small-volume viscous pancreatic secretions containing low concentrations of enzymes and bicarbonate are obtained; pancreatitis is uncommon; and (g) treatment consists of pancreatic extracts, respiratory care, and medical management of meconium ileus or small bowel obstruction (pancreatic enzymes, stool softener, oral or rectal N-acetylcysteine, and Gastrografin enemas); if this fails, surgery should be the next step.

11. *Shwachman's syndrome* is the combination of exocrine pancreatic insufficiency and hematological abnormalities (neutropenia, thrombocytopenia, anemia, and occasionally immunoglobulin deficiency) with normal sweat electrolytes. A few cases of metaphyseal chondrodysplasia and liver abnormalities have been reported.

12. *Annular pancreas* is a congenital defect in which a ring of pancreatic tissue surrounds the descending duodenum. It causes vomiting in infants and abdominal pain with incomplete obstruction of the duodenum in adults. When the "ring" is insufficiently drained, it may be the site of chronic pancreatitis and subsequent fibrosis. Plain abdominal film shows the "double-bubble" sign. The preferred treatment for symptomatic disease is bypass surgery.

13. *Ectopic pancreatic tissue* has been reported in the stomach, duodenum, jejunum, navel, spleen, gallbladder, and Meckel's diverticle.

14. *Pancreas divisum* is the most common congenital lesion of the pancreas, found in about 5% of patients at endoscopic retrograde cholangiopancreatography (ERCP). It is the result of failure of the ventral and dorsal pancreatic buds to fuse. It probably predisposes to recurrent pancreatitis because the accessory papilla draining most of the pancreas hinders pancreatic juice flow.

15. *Acute recurrent pancreatitis* has been reported in 30% of patients with type I hyperlipidemia, in 15% with type IV, and in 30–40% with type V.

16. *Acute pancreatitis* is brought about by obstruction to the outflow of pancreatic secretion, resulting in intrapancreatic activation of digestive enzymes. Per definition, there is no permanent functional damage, and the pancreas is restored to normal morphology and function after the acute episode.

17. The two most common *causes of acute pancreatitis* are *alcohol* and *gallstones*. The former may cause the development of chronic pancreatitis, which usually does not develop after episodes of acute pancreatitis induced by gallstones. Other less common causes of acute pancreatitis are hyperlipidemia (see above), trauma, hypothermia, hyperparathyroidism, vasculitis, infectious agents (mumps, coxsackie B, *Campylobacter*, *Mycoplasma*) and drugs (thiazides, furosemide, azathioprine, sulfa, tetracyclines). Acute fatty liver of pregnancy and thrombotic thrombocytopenic purpura are rare causes.

18. *Clinical features of acute pancreatitis* include (a) steady epigastric pain, often radiating to the back, usually worse when lying supine, with prominent abdominal tenderness commonly present; (b) nausea and vomiting that commonly persist for at least 24 hr, with failure of vomiting to relieve the epigastric pain; (c) body temperature elevated to 100–101°F or more; (d) development of ileus; (e) hypotension or circulatory shock in about 40% of cases; (f) jaundice in 40% of patients (results from compression of the terminal common bile duct by the inflamed pancreas); and (g) gastritis with erosions and minor mucosal bleeding caused by direct extension of the inflammation.

15   _____

19. The *diagnostic approach to suspected acute pancreatitis* considers the following: (a) other acute conditions that are easier to diagnose are excluded, e.g., perforated peptic ulcer, acute cholangitis, and mesenteric infarction; (b) levels of serum amylase rise within a few hours after onset of symptoms and return to normal within 1–2 days, but a normal serum amylase does not exclude acute pancreatitis and the magnitude of elevation does not correlate with severity of the disease or prognosis; increased serum *pancreatic isoamylase* may be found in all types of inflammatory, neoplastic, and obstructive diseases, and in gastric and small intestinal perforation; (c) amylase-creatinine clearance ratio (normal 1–4%) rises early in the course of acute pancreatitis; it is somewhat more specific than serum amylase but may also be elevated in the postoperative state, burns, diabetic ketoacidosis, and chronic renal insufficiency; (d) serum lipase levels rise within 24 hr from the onset of symptoms and remain elevated for 5–10 days; serum lipase is not more specific for acute pancreatitis than serum amylase; (e) radiological studies useful in the diagnosis of acute pancreatitis include plain abdominal film (sentinel loop and/or absence of gas in the transverse colon, the so-called "colon cut off sign"), ultrasonography (gallstones, enlarged edematous pancreas, pseudocyst, abscess), and CT (demonstrates features similar to those demonstrated by ultrasonography); and (f) ERCP is contraindicated during acute pancreatitis.

20. *Management of uncomplicated acute pancreatitis* includes (a) analgesia, usually with narcotic agents such as meperidine; (b) restoration and maintenance of intravascular volume (a significant volume may be sequestered as peripancreatic exudate); (c) NPO with nasogastric (N-G) tube; (d) hourly antacids through the N-G tube or H_2-blockers intravenously when gastric aspirate indicates bleeding; and (e) administration of a low-fat six-meal bland diet when the pain has subsided and peristalsis has returned.

21. *The management of necrotizing or prolonged pancreatitis*, when hospital course is extended or severe acute complications such as cardiovascular collapse, adult respiratory distress syndrome (ARDS), intraabdominal hemorrhage, or acute renal failure (ARF) develop, includes (a) close monitoring in an intensive care unit (ICU); (b) pressor agents when hypotension persists despite adequate IV fluids (including albumin); (c) peritoneal lavage to be repeated every 1–2 hr (for removal of pancreatic exudate); (d) consideration of emergency laparotomy for sump drainage of the necrotic pancreas and peripancreatic space, when clinical deterioration persists, especially when gallstones are suspected to be a part of the etiology; and (e) concomitantly, supportive measures to combat hypocalcemia and respiratory and renal insufficiency.

22. *Ranson's criteria for a complicated course and increased mortality risk in acute pancreatitis* are categorized as follows: (a) in acute ethanol-associated pancreatitis on admission: age over 55, WBC >16,000/mm^3, blood glucose >200 mg/dl (no history of diabetes), serum LDH >350 IU/liter, SGOT >250 IU/liter (normal up to 40); (b) in acute pancreatitis unrelated to ethanol, any time during first 48 hr after hospitalization: WBC >15,000/mm^3, blood glucose >180 mg/dl, BUN >45 mg/dl (after adequate hydration), PaO$_2$ <60 mm Hg, serum calcium <8.0 mg/dl, serum albumin <3.2 g/dl, serum LDH >600 IU/liter, SGOT or SGPT >200 IU/liter (normal up to 40).

23. *Localized complications of acute pancreatitis* are as follows: (a) *pseudocysts*: fluid collections within the pancreas or adjacent structures that occur in up to 50% of patients with severe pancreatitis; usually present as a palpable mass, at least one-half resolving spontaneously within 6 weeks; if become infected, bleed, or expand rapidly, surgical intervention is required; pseudocysts are more common with chronic pancreatitis; (b) *pancreatic ascites*: a chemical peritonitis occurring as an occasional complication of acute pancreatitis, may be massive when resulting from a break in the pancreatic duct; it is an exudate with elevated levels of amylase; when the ascites is the result of a leak in a duct, surgery is in order in patients who do not respond to conservative approach; (c) *fat necrosis*: produced by pancreatic enzymes dripping down the abdominal gutters; the adjacent transverse colon may become narrowed or obstructed, or a massive GI hemorrhage may develop when a blood vessel is invaded; (d) *splenic vein thrombosis*: may result from inflammation invading the vessel which runs along the superior margin of the pancreas; esophageal and gastric varices and splenomegaly may develop; (e) *pancreatic phlegmon*: a mass of inflamed pancreas containing patchy areas of necrosis that may be confused with a pseudocyst on ultrasonography or CT, usually subsiding within 2 weeks; should be observed for the indication of infection, thrombosis, or localized hemorrhage; and (f) *pancreatic abscess*: occurs in 2–6% of patients with acute pancreatitis, correlates with severity of the attack, should be drained surgically under antibiotic coverage (penicillin + chloramphenicol or cefoxitin); fistulas occur postoperatively in 25% of patients.

24. After recovery from *acute pancreatitis*, chances of recurrence within the next 1–2 years are 25–60%. Repeated attacks may be prevented by searching for correctable conditions, mainly gallstones (with 35–50% having another episode of acute pancreatitis within a few weeks of the first attack) but also chronic alcohol intake, hyperlipidemia, drugs, and obstruction at the ampulla of Vater.

25. When none of the conditions mentioned above is found on history, biochemical tests of the serum, or ultrasonography, ERCP should be performed about 2 weeks after recovery from *acute pancreatitis*. Recent studies have shown that nearly 60% of patients diagnosed as having idiopathic relapsing pancreatitis were found to have surgically remediable abnormalities, such as choledocholithiasis, cholelithiasis, obstruction of the pancreatic duct by calculi, strictures, small pseudocysts, or carcinoma and obstruction of the papilla Vater by fibrosis, calculi, or tumor, or pancreas divisum.

26. *Recurrent attacks of acute pancreatitis* are distinguished from acute exacerbations of chronic pancreatitis by the lack of any evidence of persistent structural or functional impairment of the gland in the former.

27. *Chronic pancreatitis* is characterized by recurrent attacks of pancreatitis, usually alcoholic in origin, which lead to progressive anatomical and functional damage to the pancreas from which it never completely recovers.

28. In 90% of patients with *chronic pancreatitis*, the etiology is chronic alcohol abuse. Other rare causes are protein malnutrition (particularly Kwashiorkor), hyperlipemia, hyperparathyroidism, and familial pancreatitis. Repeated acute attacks of gallstone pancreatitis do not progress to chronic pancreatitis.

29. *Symptoms of chronic pancreatitis* include (a) continuous or intermittent abdominal pain; (b) malabsorption with steatorrhea; and (c) diabetes mellitus.

30. In *chronic pancreatitis*, calcium is deposited in the parenchyma of the pancreas and sometimes in the ducts. *Calcifications* may be seen on plain abdominal films and CT scans.

31. *Chronic pancreatitis* may be caused by the intake of 60 g or more of alcohol daily. Most alcoholic patients already have sustained permanent structural and functional damage to the pancreas by the time of their first attack.

32. *Pain of chronic pancreatitis* is similar in character to the pain in acute pancreatitis. Some patients remain completely free of symptoms between attacks, while others complain of persistent pain (even when they refrain from drinking).

33. *Diabetes of longstanding chronic pancreatitis* can be distinguished from the common form of diabetes mellitus by the following features: (a) frequent hypoglycemic attacks; (b) a smaller requirement for insulin; (c) ineffectiveness of oral hypoglycemic agents; (d) rarity of ketoacidosis; and (e) absence of accelerated vascular disease. Most of these differences may be ascribed to low levels of glucagon in the patient with chronic pancreatitis (due to destruction of the islet cells by fibrosis).

34. In *malabsorption in chronic pancreatitis*, (a) loss of fat and protein is the main result with carbohydrate spared because amylase is also produced in the salivary glands and duodenum; (b) steatorrhea is quantitatively less than in celiac sprue; and (c) clinical evidence of fat-soluble vitamin deficiency is uncommon because absorption is largely dependent on the presence of bile.

35. The incidence of *pancreatic carcinoma* is not increased in patients with chronic pancreatitis (the rare case of hereditary pancreatitis is a possible exception).

36. In *chronic pancreatitis, the mortality rate* is 3–4% a year. About one-half of deaths are a direct result of the pancreatic disease, and the remainder are caused by acute GI bleeding, hypoglycemia, carcinomas, and complications of alcoholism.

37. Contrary to common opinion in the past, recent studies have shown that about one-half of patients with *chronic pancreatitis* also have a significant alcoholic liver disease.

38. In *chronic pancreatitis*, serum amylase and lipase concentrations are frequently normal during attacks of pain. Increased levels of these enzymes are occasionally sustained in the presence of *pseudocysts* or *pancreatic ascites*.

39. *Obstructive jaundice* may occur in 5–10% of patients with chronic pancreatitis and is ascribed to obstruction of the distal common bile duct by pancreatic fibrosis.

40. *Tests to evaluate pancreatic exocrine function* include (a) *secretin test*: measures the total output of HCO_3 in duodenal contents following IV injection of secretin; this is the most reliable test of pancreatic exocrine function; (b) endogenous stimulation for hormonal secretion, achieved by perfusion of the duodenum with amino or fatty acids or by ingesting a standard meal (e.g., *Lundh test meal*) and by measuring pancreatic secretion (using a multi-lumen tube); and (c) the *p-aminobenzoic (PABA) test or Bentiromide test*: a synthetic peptide specifically hydrolyzed by chymotrypsin is given orally; the product of hydrolysis, PABA is then conjugated in the liver and excreted in the urine to provide an indirect index of pancreatic exocrine function; this test is sensitive in advanced pancreatic insufficiency but is less useful in milder cases or when other GI or hepatic disorders coexist.

41. *Radiological diagnosis of chronic pancreatitis* includes several procedures: (a) plain abdominal film: diffuse pancreatic calcifications are demonstrated in 30% of patients; (b) ultrasonography: helpful in recognizing a pseudocyst, but the pancreas itself may appear normal even when it is actually firm and fibrotic; (c) CT can demonstrate calculi in the pancreatic duct, dilatation of the duct, and sometimes atrophy and fibrosis; pseudocyts are also demonstrated; (d) barium studies of the stomach and duodenum: not of great help in the diagnosis of chronic pancreatitis; deformities of the duodenal mucosa may result from inflammation in the adjacent pancreas and are best demonstrated on hypotonic duodenography; and (e) ERCP: useful in demonstrating ductal changes; strictures, cysts, and ductal calculi may be seen; complications include *cholangitis* (mainly in patients with preexisting obstructive jaundice) and less than 3% incidence of pancreatitis.

42. None of the radiological techniques mentioned above can distinguish *chronic pancreatitis* from *pancreatic cancer*. Cytologic examination of CT or ultrasound-guided aspirations have a sensitivity of 80% for cancer. Sometimes an open biopsy has to be performed to establish the diagnosis.

43. *Complications of chronic pancreatitis* include (a) *pancreatic pseudocysts*: encapsulated collections of fluid with high concentrations of pancreatic enzymes; may occur after episodes of acute pancreatitis, develop gradually in chronic pancreatitis, or result from trauma to the pancreas; pseudocysts are solitary in 85% of cases and may cause pain, low-grade fever, anorexia, nausea and vomiting, or signs of compression on adjacent organs (obstructive jaundice, pyloric stenosis); ultrasonography and CT scans can demonstrate the cysts, and the role of ERCP lies in the demonstration of pancreatic duct and pseudocyst anatomy immediately before scheduled surgical intervention (caution: ERCP is risky in terms of infection; antibiotic coverage is necessary, and surgical treatment of the cyst is recommended within 24 hr); about 40% of pseudocysts resolve spontaneously within 6 weeks of presumed onset, but those present for more than 6 weeks are likely to result in complications such as infection, rupture, or hemorrhage, which have a high mortality rate; rapid enlargement of a pseudocyst, verified by sonography, is an indication for surgery; (b) *pancreatic ascites*: the result of a persistent leak of pancreatic juice from a disrupted pancreatic duct or from a pseudocyst; it is painless and usually massive, and the fluid contains high amylase levels (>1000 IU/dl); (c) *common bile duct obstruction*: occurs in 5–10% of patients with chronic pancreatitis; (d) *portal and splenic vein thrombosis*: from compression by a fibrotic pancreas or a pseudocyst—occurs rarely and results in extrahepatic portal hypertension; and (e) *peptic ulcer disease*: present in about 20% of patients with chronic pancreatitis.

44. *Medical treatment of chronic pancreatitis* includes (a) abstinence from alcohol; (b) relief of pain, which usually requires the administration of narcotics; (c) a wholesome diet with moderate limitation of fat: the preferred diet should contain 3000–6000 kCal, providing 100–150 g protein and 400 g or more of carbohydrate; fat intake should begin with 50 g, increasing gradually until steatorrhea becomes clinically apparent; total parenteral nutrition (TPN) or enteral feeding may be needed for weeks to months; medium-chain triglycerides may be used to replace part of the fat in the diet; (d) replacement of pancreatic enzymes to control exocrine pancreatic insufficiency: activity of pancreatic enzymes given orally is limited due to destruction by gastric acid and dilution by gastric secretion; if the amount of steatorrhea is not reduced by 4–8 tablets of the pancreatic supplement taken just before or with the meals, an H_2-blocker, such as cimetidine 300 mg, 30 min before the meal, should be tried (note: 90% of pancreatic function has to be reduced before significant steatorrhea occurs, and enzyme preparations should be given only when they are needed, not simply because a diagnosis of chronic pancreatitis has been made); (e) with diabetes mellitus, dietary manipulations; when insulin is required, it should be administered with extreme caution due to the tendency to hypoglycemia in this disease; (f) with severe steatorrhea, when hyperoxaluria is a danger, a diet low in oxalate and long-chain triglycerides with pancreatic enzyme replacement and increased intake of calcium, which are of benefit in reducing hyperoxaluria.

45. *Surgical treatment of chronic pancreatitis* is usually attempted for relief of intractable pain. Pancreatic insufficiency is not an indication for surgery. Pain in this disease often remits spontaneously, and surgery should be postponed as long as possible. When ERCP reveals obstructed dilated pancreatic ducts, drainage surgery is recommended (pancreaticojejunostomy). When the ducts are not dilated or when disease is confined to a segment of the gland, subtotal pancreatectomy is the operation of choice. Abstinence from alcohol postoperatively is mandatory.

46. *Pancreatic carcinoma* currently represents the fourth most common cause of cancer death in males (after cancer of the lung, colon, and prostate) and the fifth in females (after breast, colon, lung, and genitalia). M:F ratio is 2:1.

47. A sixfold increase of *pancreatic cancer* has been recently reported in diabetic women but not in men. A twofold increase has been reported in cigarette smokers as compared with nonsmokers; an increased incidence has also been reported among avid coffee drinkers. However, the precise role of these and other factors in the etiology of this disease is still in need of considerable clarification.

48. *Symptoms and signs of pancreatic cancer*: (a) dull midepigastric pain, occasionally going through the back (unrelated to meals); (b) weight loss as the earliest and most common manifestation, which may be associated with anorexia, aversion to meat, a metallic taste in the mouth, diarrhea, and vomiting (the latter may signal gastric or duodenal invasion or peritoneal metastases); (c) obstructive jaundice noted in more than 50% of patients; (d) an abdominal mass palpable at the time of presentation in about 25% of patients; painless distention of the gallbladder (Courvoisier's sign) is typical but not very common; (e) depression and other mental symptoms (common); and (f) rare manifestations, including severe back pain, migratory thrombophlebitis, pruritus, acute pancreatitis, and diabetes mellitus.

49. *Diagnostic approach to pancreatic carcinoma*: (a) There is still no single diagnostic test with high sensitivity and specificity to facilitate early diagnosis of resectable and curable lesions. (b) Laboratory tests are not specific, serum alkaline phosphatase and 5-nucleotidase are elevated in about 80% of patients; SGOT, LDH, and bilirubin in about 60%; and amylase and lipase in about 17%; various serologic markers have been suggested, among them carcinoembryonic antigen (CEA), alpha-fetoprotein, parathyroid hormone, calcitonin, glucagon, insulin, C-peptide, human chorionic gonadotrophin, galactosyltransferase isoenzyme II, and elastase I, but all have a relatively low sensitivity or need further evaluation in large prospective trials. (c) When suspicion of pancreatic cancer arises, ultrasonography should be performed; it will demonstrate a mass in about 65% of cases. If the pancreas is not visualized, or atypical findings are recorded, CT should be the next diagnostic step. When CT is negative but the common bile and pancreatic ducts are dilated, an ERCP examination is warranted (it has a sensitivity of 93% for pancreatic cancer). If a large pancreatic mass is found on CT scan, ERCP or transhepatic cholangiography should be performed if bile ducts are dilated, while guided aspiration biopsy is the procedure of choice if bile ducts are not dilated. Findings on ERCP in pancreatic cancer include a solitary irregular ductal stenosis, abrupt or gradual occlusion of the main duct, displacement of Wirsung's duct, fragmentation and displacement of ductules, changes in the side branches in the vicinity of the tumor, and pooling of the contrast agent in irregular pockets of necrotic tumor mass. (d) According to recent studies, the liberal use of ERCP in patients complaining of weight loss combined with epigastric discomfort increased the rate of early detection of small pancreatic tumors with greater chance for resectability.

50. *Management of pancreatic cancer*: (a) curative resection: possible in a small minority of the patients (13% in one very large series from the Mayo Clinic (Edis A et al, Mayo Clin Proc 55:531, 1980); (b) total pancreatectomy (combined with resection of the entire duodenum, spleen, and greater omentum with subtotal gastrectomy and lymphadenectomy): the procedure of choice for patients with stages I and II of the disease as shown in recent studies (the traditional Whipple procedure should be reserved for patients with small periampullary tumors; in large nonresectable tumor masses, the "double-bypass" procedure is in order, i.e., a gastrojejunostomy to relieve duodenal obstruction and a choledochojejunostomy to relieve biliary obstruction); (c) percutaneous transhepatic stenting of the common bile duct following a transhepatic cholangiogram may be employed preoperatively to improve the clinical state of patients selected for curative resection or as a palliative procedure in jaundiced patients with large nonresectable tumors; (d) chemotherapy: 5-fluorouracil (5-FU) and other agents offer little if any improvement in survival of patients with nonresectable pancreatic malignancy; and (e) combination of megavoltage radiation and chemotherapy: has prolonged median survival from 6 to 12 months.

51. *Prognosis of pancreatic carcinoma*: less than 2% of patients survive 2 years; overall, regardless of therapy, 0.4% survive 5 years.

52. *Secretory tumors of the pancreas* are thought to arise from pluripotent stem cells in the duct epithelium called nesidioblasts, and not from islet cells. The clinical syndromes associated with these tumors result from secretion of one of the following hormones: gastrin (Zollinger–Ellison syndrome), insulin, glucagon, vasoactive intestinal peptide (VIP), somatostatin, and a few other gastroenteropancreatic peptides.

53. Pancreatic endocrine tumors or hyperplasia with secretion of one or more of the above hormones may be part of *multiple endocrine neoplasia* type I (MEN 1, Wermer's syndrome), which includes, in addition to pancreatic involvement, secretory tumors (or hyperplasia) of the pituitary and parathyroid glands.

54. The typical triad of symptoms associated with *insulinoma* includes (a) symptoms of insulin shock with fasting; (b) fasting blood sugar of less than half-normal; and (c) relief of symptoms with infusion of glucose. A plasma proinsulin value of greater than 40 fmol is diagnostic. Surgical resection is the treatment of choice.

55. In *watery diarrhea hypokalemia achlorhydria (WDHA)* syndrome, or *Verner–Morrison* syndrome, (a) VIP is assumed to be the cause of symptoms, but this is still controversial; (b) symptoms include profuse watery, secretory diarrhea and hypokalemia; (c) the tumor is malignant in 37% of patients; 20% have diffuse hyperplasia of pancreatic islets; (d) extrapancreatic tumors arising in the neural crest have been reported; (e) steroids have been shown to diminish diarrhea, but resection is the preferred treatment; and (f) the combination of streptozotocin and 5-FU has proved effective for inoperable lesions.

56. In *glucagonoma*, diabetes mellitus, weight loss and anemia are the predominant manifestations. Skin lesions resembling those seen in zinc deficiency have been reported, i.e., *migratory necrolytic erythema, atrophic glossitis,* and *stomatitis.* Glucagonomas tend to be large (usually over 3 cm). Most are malignant, and resection is the treatment of choice.

57. *Somatostatinoma* is an extremely rare secretory tumor of the pancreas. The triad of symptoms most frequently encountered includes gallstones, diabetes, and diarrhea with steatorrhea.

6
The Biliary Tract

1. The *gallbladder capacity* is 30–50 ml. Wall thickness while fasting is up to 3.5 mm. Maximal diameter of common bile duct is 7–8 mm in intravenous cholangiography (IVC) or ultrasonography, 10–11 mm on ERCP or percutaneous transhepatic cholangiography (PTC).

2. The *common bile duct* is 3 inches (7.5 cm) long.

3. *Functions of Oddi* are (a) regulation of bile flow to the intestine; (b) prevention of bile reflux into the pancreatic duct; and (c) prevention of reflux of intestinal contents into biliary and pancreatic ducts.

4. The *sphincter of Oddi* maintains a positive pressure of 3–10 mm Hg in the common hepatic duct.

5. After stimulation with *CCK*, the gallbladder empties 50% of its contents in 12 min, 75% within 30 min.

6. *"Biliary pain"* is not colicky, is in the RUQ or epigastrium, and is common between 2 and 6 a.m.

7. *Pain from stones in the gallbladder* usually lasts less than 4 hr, with minimal radiation to the back; there is no vomiting.

8. In *acute cholecystitis*, the pain is more prolonged. When a stone

8

migrates to the common bile duct, prolonged pain and vomiting are common.

9. With prolonged pain, severe back pain, and profuse vomiting, *gallstone pancreatitis* should be excluded.

10. *Cholangitis* is rare in malignant obstruction of the common bile duct.

11. There is no convincing evidence for the association of *gallstone disease* and *coronary artery disease.* Cholecystectomy should not be performed in an effort to treat coronary artery disease.

12. *Oral contraceptives* promote gallstone formation through progesterone (increased cholesterol saturation).

13. *Low-fiber diet* contributes to gallstone formation (increased cholesterol secretion in bile).

14. *TPN* contributes to gallstone formation (stasis in gallbladder while fasting).

15. First-degree relatives of *gallstone patients* run a higher (2:1) risk of the development of gallstones.

16. *Cholesterol stones* comprise 70–80% of bile stones in the Western world. After the sixth decade of life, *pigment stones* become more common.

17. *Bile acid pool* is reduced in size in gallstone disease—it may be the primary defect in stone formation. Elevated *HMG–CoA reductase,* which accelerates cholesterol production, and depressed levels of *7-alpha-hydroxylase,* which reduces synthesis of primary bile acids, have also been demonstrated.

18. Clinical settings with increased incidence of *pigment stones* include hemolysis, cirrhosis, and aging.

19. After resection of a significant portion of the ileum or the administration of *cholestyramine,* gallstones are the result of reduced bile acid pool. *Ileostomy* increases gallstone prevalence to 24% (from 11.6% in the general population).

20. *Obese* patients secrete more cholesterol in their bile (overproduction in the liver? overproduction in adipose tissue? increased intestinal absorption?).

21. *Chenodeoxycholic acid (CDA)* reduces cholesterol in bile through decreased intestinal absorption, decreased production, and decreased secretion in bile.

22. The potential *hepatotoxic effect of CDA* is probably the result of its metabolism by intestinal bacteria to *lithocholic acid*.

23. *CDA* should be administered at night when bile salts are sequestered in the gallbladder and the bile acid pool is reduced.

24. Factors that reduce the chance for successful *medical therapy of gallstones* include (a) the presence of pigment stones; (b) large stones; (c) calcification; (d) obesity; and (e) recurrence.

25. *Complications of CDA* include (a) diarrhea (in 40% of patients when more than 15 mg/kg is given); (b) elevated SGOT in 31% of patients; (c) clinically significant liver disease in 3%; and (d) 10% increase in LDL cholesterol.

26. *Ursodeoxycholic acid* is as effective as CDA in gallstone dissolution, but a lower effective dose can be used (8 mg/kg vs. 12–15 mg/kg); diarrhea is uncommon, and there is no heptotoxicity.

27. Seventy-five percent of patients with *acute cholecystitis* had prior episodes of biliary pain.

28. *Acalculous cholecystitis* comprises 10% of acute cholecystitis. In 90% of patients with acute cholecystitis, stones are present.

29. *Predisposing factors to acalculous cholecystitis* include starvation, immobilization (postoperative, in patients hospitalized with TPN, CVA, trauma, burns), *Salmonella*, and cholera carriers.

30. Mild to moderate jaundice is present in 25% of patients with *acute cholecystitis* (small stones passing from gallbladder to common bile duct?).

31. *Amylase* and *lipase* are elevated in 25% of patients with *acute cholecystitis*. SGOT is occasionally elevated.

32. The *prevalence of gallstones* in the general population is 11.6%; in *diabetics* over 20 years of age, 30%.

33. The gallbladder is palpable in one-third of patients with *acute cholecystitis*.

34. An attack of *acute cholecystitis* usually lasts 7–10 days. Earlier resolution is not uncommon.

35. *HIDA isotopic scans* are sensitive for both calculous and acalculous cholecystitis.

36. Antimicrobials are useless in early stages of *acute cholecystitis* when pain resolves with meperidine (Demerol) and atropine and there is no fever or leukocytosis.

37. When the clinical picture of *acute cholecystitis* is more dramatic, management includes N-G tube, IV fluids, antimicrobial agents (cephazolin or ampicillin for mild cases, mezlocillin or cefotaxim + gentamycin + metronidazole for severe cases), and early surgery.

38. In critically ill patients, *cholecystostomy* is the preferred surgical procedure.

39. *Mortality from acute cholecystitis* is 5%; in patients over age 70, 15%; and in diabetes mellitus, 20%.

40. Abdominal pain is the most common presentation of *gallbladder empyema* (94%).

41. Most authorities agree with a nonsurgical approach to *asymptomatic gallstones*.

42. A *surgical approach toward gallstones* is supported by the presence of (a) nonfunctioning gallbladder; (b) stones larger than 2.5 cm;

and (c) porcelain gallbladder (carries a higher tendency for carcinoma).

43. In patients with *gallstones*, plain films of the abdomen demonstrate stones in 15% of patients.

44. Increased incidence of colonic adenomata has been found 10 years after *cholecystectomy* (Mannes AG et al, Gut 26:863, 1984).

45. *Sludge* is not an indication for cholecystectomy.

46. *After cholecystectomy*, (a) bile salt pool decreases in size; (b) the frequency of enterohepatic circulation increases; and (c) there is an increased percentage of secondary bile acids in the bile.

47. Fifteen percent of patients with *gallbladder stones* have stones in the common bile duct (CBD); the association increases with age; and 95% of patients with CBD stones have gallbladder stones.

48. *Resting pressure in CBD* is 10–15 cm H_2O; in complete obstruction: 25–40 cm H_2O. Bile flow stops when pressure is over 30 cm H_2O.

49. *Alkaline phosphatase* is elevated in biliary obstruction due to increased synthesis in canalicular membranes with regurgitation into the sinusoids.

50. *Alkaline phosphatase* may be elevated even in the presence of an insignificant biliary obstruction, whereas the degree of bilirubin elevation is proportional to the extent of obstruction.

51. The development of *secondary biliary cirrhosis* is a slow process—about 5 years in untreated choledocholithiasis—but may be accelerated in an unrelieved malignant obstruction (3–4 months).

52. In *choledocholithiasis*, bilirubin rarely exceeds 12 mg/dl, and alkaline phosphatase uncommonly exceeds five times normal. In malignant obstruction, both can exceed these values.

53. *Bile duct obstruction* is required for the development of cholangitis.

54. *Cholangitis* is common in choledocholithiasis, almost universal in posttraumatic stricture, but rare in neoplastic obstruction.

55. *Common bacteria in infected bile* are *E. coli, Klebsiella, Pseudomonas, Enterococcus,* and *Proteus.* Accompanying anaerobes present in 15% of cases are *Bacteroides fragilis* and *Clostridium perfringens.*

56. *Treatment of acute cholangitis* involves the same antimicrobial therapy as in acute cholecystitis. Severe or refractory cases may require *endoscopic sphincterotomy* or surgery.

57. *Complications of CBD stones* are (a) cholangitis; (b) pancreatitis; (c) hepatic abscess; and (d) cirrhosis.

58. Once *CBD stones* have been demonstrated, they should be surgically removed at the earliest convenience.

59. *Papillary dysfunction* proved by manometry (through an ERCP) has been found in fewer than 1% of patients after cholecystectomy and in 14% of those complaining of abdominal pain after cholecystectomy (Bar-Meir S et al, Hepatology 4:328, 1984).

60. *Biliary dyskinesia* is a controversial entity. It has recently been defined as high resting pressure in the sphincter of Oddi with change in the direction of propagation of the phasic contractions in a patient with (a) intermittent RUQ pain; (b) intermittent mild elevation of SGOT; and c) normal ERCP (Meshkinpour H et al, Gastroenterology 87:759, 1984).

61. *Indications for CBD exploration* in gallbladder surgery include (a) history of cholangitis; (b) recent jaundice; (c) history of pancreatitis; (d) dilated CBD; and (e) palpable stones in CBD.

62. Patients with deep *obstructive jaundice and cholangitis* are susceptible to *ARF.*

63. *Gallstones* do not cause dyspepsia.

64. *Sonographic criteria for gallstones* are (a) echogenicity; (b) the casting of shadows; and (c) movement with change of position.

65. Differential diagnosis of *gas in the biliary tract* includes chole-dochoduodenal or cholecystoduodenal fistula, incompetent sphincter of Oddi, and anaerobic infection.

66. In *gallstone ileus*, the stone is usually larger than 2.5 cm.

67. Differential diagnosis of *hemobilia* includes (a) trauma; (b) post-ERCP; (c) post-liver biopsy (rare); (d) aneurysm of hepatic artery; (e) carcinoma; and (f) ascariasis.

68. *Postcholecystectomy syndrome* is common in patients operated on for dyspeptic symptoms erronously ascribed to gallstones.

69. In a series of 16,700 postcholecystectomy patients (by Glenn), *retained stones* were found in 1.1%.

70. Of those patients with *retained common duct calculi* after biliary surgery, one-half will become symptomatic within 5 years.

71. *Cholangitis* within 2 years of surgery is the common symptom of postoperative *stricture of the CBD*.

72. Antibiotic coverage is necessary before ERCP or THC when a *stricture* is suspected.

73. *Sphincterotomy*, or papillotomy, is the treatment of choice for *retained stones* after cholecystectomy.

74. Two years after sphincterotomy, a 25% reduction in length of the surgical cut was found, but low resting pressure gradient between CBD and duodenum was maintained (Geenen JE et al, Gastroenterology 87:754, 1984).

75. *Complications of sphincterotomy* include morbidity (10%), mainly bleeding, pancreatitis, perforation, and cholangitis. Mortality occurs in 1.2% of cases.

76. In *external biliary fistula*, the preferred replacement of fluid and electrolyte losses is to return bile by drinking or N-G tube. If impossible, correction of fluid and electrolyte imbalance should be sought.

77. The most common fixed filling defect in the gallbladder is a *cholesterol polyp.*

78. The most common malignant tumor of the gallbladder is *scirrhous adenocarcinoma.*

79. As many as 80–85% of patients with *gallbladder carcinoma* have gallstones.

80. *Biliary tract carcinoma* is associated with ulcerative colitis; choledochal cyst; Caroli's disease; workers in rubber, automotive, wood, and chemical industries; and *Clonorchis sinensis.*

81. The *5-year survival in gallbladder carcinoma* is less than 1%.

82. Colectomy does not prevent the higher tendency for *biliary tract carcinoma* in ulcerative colitis.

83. *Nasobiliary or percutaneous drainage* is recommended for 7–10 days before surgery in *obstructive cholangiocarcinoma.*

84. Fluctuant jaundice is typical of *ampullary carcinoma.*

7
The Liver

1. On physical examination, the normal *span of the liver* as measured by percussion in the right midclavicular line is 12–15 cm. It is the largest organ in the body.

2. *Riedel's lobe* is a common anatomical abnormality. This downward tonguelike projection of the right lobe is more common in women than in men. It does not cause symptoms, and treatment is not required.

3. *Liver cells (hepatocytes)* comprise about 60% of the liver mass. Their life-span is about 150 days.

4. The *excretory system* of the liver begins with the bile canaliculi, which drain into thin-walled terminal bile ducts (known also as ductules, cholangioles, or canals of Hering); these terminate in larger (interlobular) bile ducts in the portal spaces.

5. The following types of cells are found in the sinusoidal wall: (a) endothelial cells; (b) Kupffer cells; (c) lipocytes (Ito cells), which probably represent undifferentiated mesenchymal cells or resting fibroblasts; and (d) Pit cells, which contain granules and may have an endocrine function.

6. A palpable or audible *friction rub* over the liver is usually attributable to a tumor, a recent biopsy, or perihepatitis.

7. A *venous hum* may be heard between the umbilicus and the xiphisternum in portal hypertension.

8. An *arterial murmur* over the liver may indicate a primary liver cancer or acute alcoholic hepatitis.

9. An increase of *urobilinogen in the urine* is found when hepatocellular function is inadequate to reexcrete all the bilirubin absorbed from the intestine. Thus, urinary urobilinogen is an index of hepatocellular dysfunction.

10. *Cholesterol* is synthesized in the liver, small intestine, and other tissues, from acetate. Hepatic synthesis is inhibited by cholesterol feeding and by fasting. Synthesis is increased by a biliary fistula, bile duct ligation, or an intestinal lymph fistula. The rate-limiting step is the conversion of hydroxymethylglutaryl–CoA(hMG-CoA) to mevalonate. Esterification is carried out in plasma by the enzyme lecithin cholesterol acyltransferase (LCAT), which is synthesized in the liver.

11. *Cholesterol, phospholipids,* and *triglycerides* are synthesized in the liver but are insoluble in water and cannot exist in plasma in free solution. Lipoproteins are involved in lipid transport. Four groups of lipoproteins are recognized: (a) high-density lipoproteins (HDL): migrate with alpha$_1$-globulin on electrophoresis; (b) low-density lipoproteins (LDL): migrate with beta-globulins; (c) very-low-density lipoproteins (VLDL); and (d) chylomicrons (large, triglyceride-rich particles originating in the gut and appearing in plasma after ingestion of a fatty meal).

12. *Bile salts* (a) take part in emulsification of dietary fat; (b) probably have some role in the mucosal phase of absorption; (c) assist in pancreatic lipolysis; (d) release GI hormones; (e) may contribute to the pruritus of cholestasis when levels are elevated in the serum; and (f) are responsible for the secretion of conjugated bilirubin in the urine.

13. *Serum bile acid levels* reflect the fraction reabsorbed from the

intestine that escaped extraction during its first passage through
the liver. Both hepatocellular and cholestatic jaundice may be associated with elevated serum bile acid levels.

14. Some of the *amino acids* derived from the diet and from tissue
breakdown are transaminated or deaminated in the liver to ke-
toacids, which are metabolized by many pathways. Others are
metabolized to ammonia and urea.

15. In liver failure, *aromatic amino acids* (tyrosine, phenylalanine,
tryptophan) increase in the serum due to failure of deamination.
Branched-chain aminoacids (BCAAs) are decreased due to increased
catabolism in skeletal muscle.

16. Liver disease is associated with failure to maintain *serum albumin* values, whereas immunoglobulins tend to increase. The reason is that the former is synthesized by liver cells, while the latter
is synthesized by immunocytes.

17. *Alkaline phosphatase* synthesis is increased in any disorder that
interferes with bile flow, whether intrahepatic or extrahepatic. With
a serum half-life of 7 days, it tends to remain elevated after the
serum bilirubin has returned to normal. In cholestatic jaundice,
levels are usually four times the upper limit of normal, while in
hepatocellular jaundice, they are less. Values may be increased (up
to 50% above the upper limit of the norm) after the fifth decade of
life.

18. *Serum 5-nucleotidase* level is normal in bone disease and raised
in hepatobiliary conditions, especially cholestatic jaundice.

19. *Gamma-glutamyl transpeptidase* is an enzyme found in many tissues. It does not reflect one specific hepatic function, and serum
values are increased in both cholestasis and hepatocellular disease.
It is used to confirm whether a raised serum alkaline phosphatase
is of hepatobiliary origin. It is also used to screen for alcohol abuse
when serum levels are raised.

20. *Glutamic oxaloacetic transaminase (GOT), or aspartate transaminase,* is a mitochondrial enzyme; its serum levels may rise to very high values in hepatocellular necrosis. *Glutamic pyruvic transaminase (GPT), or alanine transaminase* is a cytosol enzyme. Its increase in the serum is more specific for liver damage than is SGOT. The absolute values of SGOT and SGPT do not correlate with the degree of liver damage in *viral hepatitis.* Very high levels may be seen, not only in acute viral hepatitis but in early stages of acute choledocholithiasis as well. Values of these enzymes in cirrhosis vary from low to very high, being particularly high in *chronic active hepatitis.* A ratio of SGOT to SGPT greater than 2 is useful in diagnosing *alcoholic hepatitis* and *alcoholic cirrhosis.*

21. *Lactic dehydrogenase (LDH)* is a relatively insensitive index of hepatocellular injury.

22. Recent studies reported on other *liver enzymes* that may be of possible diagnostic value: (a) aldolase B for hepatocellular necrosis; (b) fructose 1,6-diphosphatase for piecemeal necrosis; (c) creatine phosphokinase for biliary obstruction; and (d) alpha$_2$-macroglobin serum levels—high in mechanical biliary obstruction but not in cholestatic hepatitis. All these reports are preliminary and need further investigation.

23. One recent study has reported on *indocyanine green* clearance as an early indicator of hepatic dysfunction following trauma (Gottlieb ME et al, Arch Surg 119:264, 1984).

24. *Percutaneous needle biopsy of the liver* is a procedure with low incidence of complications but should always be regarded as potentially risky. Most biopsy-induced hematomas probably go undetected. The incidence of hematomas detectable by radionuclide scanning or ultrasonography is 2.3%. They may cause fever, rises in SGOT and SGPT, and right upper quadrant tenderness. Other complications include pleuritis, perihepatitis, pneumothorax, intraperitoneal hemorrhage (extremely rare in nonjaundiced, most common in severe hepatocellular disease, uncommon in cholestatic jaundice after vitamin K therapy), biliary peritonitis (may seal spontaneously or require surgical drainage; biopsy should be avoided when dilated intrahepatic ducts are identified by ultrasonography), hemobilia, and transient septicemia. In a review of more than 23,000 needle biopsies performed during the late 1960s, mortality was found to be 0.017%. It is probably even lower today with elaboration of the needle and technique and with better definition of indications and contraindications (see Nos. 25 and 26).

25. Prothrombin time and platelet count should always be done before needle *biopsy of the liver*. Biopsy should not be performed if prothrombin time is more than 3 sec increased over control, and platelet count should exceed 80,000. Vitamin K (10 mg IM) should be administered for a period of 2 days to jaundiced patients. Tense ascites, hydatid cyst, suspected hemangioma, right empyema, right subphrenic abscess, and deep hepatocellular jaundice are *contraindications to percutaneous liver biopsy*.

26. *Indications for needle liver biopsy* include: (a) jaundice, when the diagnosis is difficult; (b) cirrhosis and portal hypertension; (c) alcoholic liver injury; (d) chronic hepatitis; (e) suspected drug-related liver disease; (f) unexplained hepatomegaly or unexplained abnormalities of liver function; (g) infective and other systemic diseases (a portion of the biopsy should be cultured when biopsy is done for a suspected infective process); (h) storage diseases; and (i) screening of relatives of patients with familial diseases.

27. *Guided-needle liver biopsy* under control of sonography or CT facilitates the diagnosis of focal lesions, such as primary tumors of the liver, metastatic tumors of the liver, and simple cysts of the liver.

28. Lebrec and associates recently reported on 1000 *transjugular liver biopsies* in patients in whom percutaneous biopsies were contraindicated mainly because of bleeding tendency. Eight hundred biopsy specimens were satisfactory, one fatal perforation of the liver occurred (Lebrec D et al, Gastroenterology 83:338, 1982).

29. *Causes of anemia in chronic liver disease* are (a) increased plasma volume (especially in portal hypertension with cirrhosis); (b) GI bleeding from varices; (c) bleeding from disturbed blood coagulation; (d) hypersplenism; (e) extrasplenic hemolysis in patients with alcoholic liver disease who also have hypercholesterolemia (Zieve's syndrome); and (f) rarely, a Coomb's positive hemolytic anemia seen in chronic active hepatitis and in primary biliary cirrhosis.

30. *Splenectomy* is not recommended in hypersplenism of chronic liver disease because the response of the RBCs is disappointing and mortality is high; also, in patients with portal hypertension it may be followed by splenic and portal vein thrombosis. Splenectomy should be performed only when clinical suffering from leukopenia or thrombocytopenia occurs.

31. *Bleeding in hepatocellular failure* is caused by (a) defective synthesis of vitamin K-dependent clotting factors II, VII, IX, and X and factor V, which is also synthesized in the liver (vitamin K is not absorbed due to insufficient bile salt secretion); (b) cell necrosis, which may lead to activation of hemostasis and disseminated intravascular coagulation (DIC) with fibrinolysis (consumptive coagulopathy can follow); and (c) defective clearance of activated factors, which may lead to DIC as well.

32. The *prothrombin time (PT)* and/or *partial thromboplastin time (PTT)* before and after administration of 10 mg vitamin K IM are the most satisfactory tests for a coagulation defect in patients with hepatobiliary disease. PT is also a most sensitive indication of the presence of hepatocellular necrosis and of prognosis.

33. In *hemolysis*, the healthy liver has a large capacity to handle the bilirubin load; even in massive hemolysis, serum bilirubin rises only to about 2–3 mg/dl. If in patients with hemolysis serum bilirubin values are greater than 4–5 mg/dl, there is probably an additional factor of hepatocellular dysfunction.

34. In *Hodgkin's disease,* hepatic involvement occurs in about 70% of cases. A multitude of parenchymal lesions have been described on biopsy, ranging from lymphocytic infiltration to focal necrosis. It is unusual for a needle biopsy of the liver to demonstrate Hodgkin's tissue if a radionuclide scan is normal.

35. In *myeloproliferative disorders,* portal hypertension may occur as a result of (a) thrombosis of the portal vein, splenic vein, or hepatic artery; (b) infiltrative lesions in the portal tracts or sinusoids; and (c) increased portal blood flow through the enlarged spleen.

36. *Plain films of the abdomen* for diagnosis of hepatobiliary disorders have been ignored in recent years. However, they may reveal gallstones, a calcified gallbladder wall, or emphysematous cholecystitis. *Gas in the biliary tree* may be due to (a) a spontaneous or postoperative biliary fistula; (b) incompetent sphincter of Oddi (as a result of gallstones or sphincterotomy); or (c) gas-gangrene infection (emphysematous cholecystitis).

37. *Oral cholecystography (OCG)* can be used to diagnose radiolucent gallstones and to evaluate gallbladder function, but it has chiefly been replaced by ultrasonography, which is now the initial diagnostic procedure for suspected gallstone disease. When there is a strong clinical suspicion of cholelithiasis or cholecystitis and the sonogram is normal, OCG can still be useful to exclude an isolated calculus in the cystic duct, which may be missed by sonography.

38. *Intravenous cholangiography (IVC)* has been largely replaced by ultrasonography and radionuclide studies for evaluation of acute cholecystitis, since the biliary system does not opacify adequately and tomography is necessary in a large number of patients. In addition, there is a false-negative rate of 17–45% in detecting chronic cholecystitis and cholelithiasis. An IVC that suggests partial obstruction by reason of delayed opacification generally requires further confirmation by direct cholangiography (PTC or ERCP) (see Nos. 43 and 44 and Chapter 5).

39. *Ultrasonography* is mainly used to detect focal lesions in the liver or to confirm suspected biliary tract disease. It is possible to distinguish among solid tumors, cysts, and abscesses, but false-positive and false-negative findings do occur. Because of its ease of application, sonography has become the preferred screening technique for suspected space-occupying lesions of the liver and for detecting biliary tract pathology. Endoscopic ultrasound probes, which facilitate the study of small lesions in the biliary tree (such as retained bile duct stones), are in the process of development.

40. *Radionuclide scintigraphy* in hepatobiliary disease is useful in (a) delineating size, location, and contour of the liver as well as uniformity of colloid distribution and the presence of "cold" lesions in the liver (^{99m}Tc); (b) determining the presence of hepatocellular disease by inhomogeneity of colloid distribution and by relatively increased activity in the spleen and bone marrow; (c) evaluating space-occupying lesions as small as 1–2 cm; (d) assessing cystic duct patency in suspected acute cholecystitis (by radiotracers that undergo hepatobiliary excretion, such as labeled N-substituted aminodiacetates, IDA group); (e) evaluating the biliary system after surgery or trauma, e.g., in suspected bile leak or fistula (IDA); (f) evaluating congenital biliary anomalies such as biliary atresia or choledochal cyst (IDA); and (g) evaluating a liver transplant (see No. 218).

41. *Cholescintigraphy (IDA)* as a means of detecting cystic duct obstruction is the preferred diagnostic technique in *suspected acute cholecystitis*.

42. *Computed tomography (CT)* of the liver and biliary tract has its main application in the diagnosis of focal lesions, such as tumors or abscesses, but it can also provide information on the nature of diffuse liver disease (hemochromatosis, glycogenosis, diffuse steatosis). CT imaging is improved when performed with contrast media. Intravenous injection of an emulsion of ethiodized oil has recently been shown to permit the detection of lesions as small as 1 cm in diameter.

43. *Endoscopic retrograde cholangiopancreatography (ERCP)* is probably the most sensitive technique for detecting stones and tumors of the common duct. It is an excellent technique for evaluating patients with (a) either intrahepatic or extrahepatic jaundice, when the latter is suspected; (b) symptoms without jaundice after biliary tract surgery; (c) other abnormal tests suggesting biliary tract disease (such as common bile duct dilatation suggested by ultrasonography); and (d) known or suspected choledocholithiasis who are potential candidates for endoscopic sphincterotomy. (For the use of ERCP in pancreatic disease, see Chapter 5.)

44. *Percutaneous transhepatic cholangiography (PTC)* is a relatively simple and safe procedure. It permits direct visualization of the biliary tract in order to detect the site and nature of obstruction in patients with suspected obstructive jaundice. As opposed to ERCP, which outlines the distal portion of an obstruction, PTC can define the proximal extent of the blockage. PTC is also indicated when there is a need for delineation of the anatomy of the biliary tract after surgery, particularly after choledochojejunal anastomosis. It is also useful in determining the patency of the ductal system in sclerosing cholangitis. By providing access to the obstructed biliary system, PTC permits external or internal drainage of bile, which is usually performed either for decompression before surgery or as a substitute for surgical decompression of a biliary tract obstruction by an inoperable tumor.

45. *Nuclear magnetic resonance (NMR)* imaging of the liver is still in a developmental stage, but preliminary observations seem promising, especially for demonstrating hepatomas and other tumors and for differentiating among various parenchymal diseases.

46. In *acute hepatocellular failure* due to such causes as viral hepatitis, jaundice parallels the extent of liver cell damage. But in chronic hepatic failure (e.g., cirrhosis) jaundice may be absent or mild; when present, it indicates active parenchymal disease and carries a poor prognosis.

47. In *hepatocellular failure*, hyperkinetic circulation (from an unknown cause) is manifested by flushed extremities, bounding pulse, capillary pulsation, increased skin and splenic blood flow, and increased cardiac output.

48. In *hepatocellular failure*, reduced oxygen saturation and cyanosis are common. This is probably due to intrapulmonary shunting through microscopic arteriovenous fistulas. The most profound cyanosis and clubbing are associated with chronic active hepatitis and long-standing cirrhosis.

49. In *active advanced cirrhosis*, about one-third of patients show a continuous low-grade fever. It is more frequent in alcoholics.

50. The *failing liver* is unable to convert ammonia to urea, but the reserve capacity of synthesis is great and blood urea levels fall only in a very advanced state or in fulminant hepatitis.

51. *Serum albumin* level falls in proportion to the degree and duration of *hepatocellular failure*. The same is true for other proteins such as prothrombin (prolonged PT is not restored to normal by vitamin K therapy) and other blood factors.

52. *Skin changes in chronic liver failure* include (a) spider angiomas, which may disappear with improving hepatic function or when blood pressure falls; (b) white spots on arms and buttocks on cooling the skin; (c) palmar erythema (also seen in rheumatoid arthritis, pregnancy, chronic febrile disease, chronic leukemia, thyrotoxicosis); and (d) white nails.

53. *Endocrine changes in chronic hepatocellular failure* include (a) diminished libido and potency; (b) sterility (in advanced cirrhosis); (c) loss of secondary sexual hair; (d) testicular atrophy; (e) erratic, diminished, or absent menstruation; (f) atrophy of breasts and uterus; and (g) gynecomastia and other features of feminization (more common in alcoholic liver disease).

54. *Management of chronic hepatocellular failure* consists of the following symptomatic measures: (a) continued bed rest while improvement is maintained; (b) diet containing 80–100 g protein and 2500 cal; (c) abstention from alcohol (one glass of wine or beer daily is allowed in nonalcoholic chronic liver disease); (d) Hb level kept above 10 g/dl; and (e) avoidance of sedatives. If the need arises, oxazepam, which has a normal disposition in hepatic failure, may be the drug of choice.

55. The three types of *hepatic encephalopathy* are (a) *chronic portal sytemic encephalopathy (PSE)* with an etiology of portal-systemic shunting or increased dietary protein intake (survival rate: 100%, with proper treatment); (b) *cirrhosis with encephalopathy* precipitated by diuretics, hemorrhage, diarrhea and vomiting, paracentesis, surgery, infection, sedatives, or alcohol excess (survival rate: 70–80%); and (c) *encephalopathy in acute liver failure,* caused by acute viral hepatitis, alcoholic hepatitis, or drug overdose (survival rate: about 20%).

56. *Symptoms of PSE* are (a) inversion of sleep pattern; (b) apathy and slowness; (c) personality changes (childishness, irritability); (d) intellectual deterioration ranging from slight impairment of organic mental function to gross confusion; (e) slurred and slow speech; and (f) stupor and coma, which represent advanced stage of encephalopathy.

57. *Flapping tremor (asterixis)* is the most characteristic neurological abnormality in PSE. It is caused by impaired inflow of joint and other afferent information to the brainstem.

58. *Electroencephalographic (EEG) changes in PSE* appear early but are nonspecific. These include slowing of the frequency from the normal alpha range of 8–13 cycles/sec to the delta range of less than 4 cycles/sec.

59. *Ammonium* is derived from the nitrogenous contents of the intestine by bacterial action and is present in high concentration in portal blood. It is metabolized by the liver to urea. The question of whether a raised blood ammonium level in hepatic coma represents a toxic causative factor or is merely a nonspecific indicator of disturbed brain metabolism remains unresolved.

60. *Blood ammonia levels* usually corelate with either severity of encephalopathy or depth of coma, but in 10% of patients values are in the normal range regardless of depth of coma. After portocaval shunts, levels may be raised when no signs of encephalopathy are present. The level does not correlate with prognosis.

61. Recent studies indicate that levels of *ammonia in erythrocytes* are a better index of PSE than are blood ammonia levels.

62. *Cerebrospinal fluid (CSF) glutamine level* is a sensitive index of PSE.

63. *Alkalosis* is common in *PSE* due to the following: (a) toxic stimulation of the respiratory center by ammonia; (b) administration of alkali such as citrate in transfusions; and (c) hypokalemia precipitated by treatment with diuretics. Alkalosis increases ammonium toxicity by increased transfer of ionized ammonia across cell membranes.

64. *Hypoglycemia* is rare in chronic liver disease but may complicate fulminant hepatitis (see No. 72). The failing liver fails to metabolize insulin and glucagon adequately.

65. *GI bleeding triggers PSE* through the large protein contents in the intestine, the depression of hepatocellular function by anemia, and the reduction in liver blood flow.

66. *Surgical procedures* are poorly tolerated by patients with advanced liver failure, since remaining hepatic function is depressed by blood loss, anesthesia, and shock.

67. A large *protein meal* or *severe constipation* may precipitate coma in advanced liver disease.

68. *Prognosis in PSE* depends on the extent of liver cell failure. In cirrhosis, such findings as ascites, jaundice, and low serum albumin are indicators of poor prognosis, as they all represent liver failure.

69. *Child's classification* of prognosis in hepatocellular disease is based on the following parameters: the presence of ascites and encephalopathy, nutritional status, serum bilirubin and albumin levels, and PT. One-year survival is around 70% for patients in grade A or B and 30% in grade C.

70. *Management of PSE* includes (a) identification and elimination of precipitating factors; (b) limitation of dietary protein to 40 g; (c) avoidance of nitrogen-containing drugs (e.g., ammonium chloride, urea); (d) 1–2 semisolid bowel movements daily ensured by lactulose 10–30 ml tid; (e) maintenance of caloric and fluid and electrolyte balance; and (f) neomycin 1–1.5 g qid, recommended especially in acute hepatic coma; metronidazole 0.2 g qid has been shown to have an additive effect. Experimental therapeutic modalities that may be employed when symptoms worsen despite the above regimen include BCAAs, bromocriptine 15 mg/day, and liver transplantation (see No. 218).

71. The mechanism of action of *lactulose in PSE* is uncertain. It is broken down by bacteria in the cecum to lactic acid and acetic acid. Fecal pH drops. Changes in conditions are created that favor the growth of lactose-fermenting organisms over ammonia formers, but clinical improvement after the administration of lactulose precedes these changes in bacterial flora. The decreased pH value reduces the ionization of NH_4 (unabsorbed) to NH_3 (absorbed), but fecal ammonia is not increased by lactulose.

72. *Acute (fulminant) hepatic failure* is a clinical syndrome resulting from massive necrosis of liver cells or from sudden and severe impairment of liver function. There should be no evidence of preceding liver disease. Possible etiologies include viral hepatitis, i.e., A, B, non-A–non-B (NANB); drugs, e.g., paracetamol and halothane; and the fatty liver of pregnancy. Survival is 12–20% if deep coma is reached. Advanced age and the coexistence of other diseases worsen the prognosis. Those who survive seldom develop chronic liver disease. Causes of death are bleeding, respiratory and circulatory failure, cerebral edema, renal failure, infection, hypoglycemia, and pancreatitis (see also No. 136).

73. *Cerebral edema* is a major factor in the mortality of acute hepatic failure. Mannitol has been shown to have a significant therapeutic value. Steroids have no proven value.

74. There is no well-founded scientific evidence showing therapeutic benefits of *BCAAs, extracorporal assists* (e.g., hemodialysis or charcoal hemoperfusion), or hepatocyte transplantation in *acute (fulminant) hepatic failure.*

75. *Ascites in portal hypertension* results from the following contributing factors: (a) both elevated portal venous pressure and hypoalbuminemia (leading to decreased colloid osmotic pressure); (b) most likely increased hepatic lymph production; and (c) sodium retention (either as a primary renal defect or secondary to low effective intravascular volume).

76. *Pleural effusion* is common among cirrhotic patients with ascites; it is caused by defects in the diaphragm permitting ascites to pass into the pleural cavity. It is right-sided in about two-thirds of cases.

77. *Peripheral edema* commonly follows the ascites in portal hypertension; it is the result of hypoproteinemia and of functional inferior vena cava block by ascitic fluid.

78. The *fluid in ascites of portal hypertension is a transudate*. Protein concentration exceeding 2 g/dl suggests infection, obstruction to the hepatic veins (Budd–Chiari syndrome), or pancreatic ascites.

79. *Spontaneous bacterial peritonitis (SBP)* (a) develops in about 8% of cirrhotic patients with ascites, more commonly in decompensated cirrhosis and in alcoholics; (b) should be suspected if the condition of a patient with a known cirrhosis shows sudden deterioration, particularly encephalopathy; (c) may be associated with fever, local abdominal pain, and tenderness and leukocytosis; (d) is not conclusively established by an ascites WBC count exceeding 500/mm³ of which at least 75% are polymorphs, but this finding is sufficiently alarming to merit antibiotic therapy; (e) is indicated with high specifity (100%) by a low ascitic fluid pH (below 7.32), but this measure has a low sensitivity (25%) as an indicator of bacterial peritonitis; (f) is most commonly caused by *Escherichia coli*, but streptococci and mixed infections do occur; (g) is treated by systemic administration of antimicrobial agents according to the sensitivity of the organism cultured from the ascitic fluid; and (h) carries a poor prognosis when accociated with acute alcoholic hepatitis, serum bilirubin above 8 mg/dl, and serum creatinine above 2.1 mg/dl.

80. *Dr. Sheila Sherlock's protocol for the management of ascites in portal hypertension* includes (a) bed rest; (b) a low-sodium diet (22 mEq/day); (c) restriction of fluid intake to 1 liter/day; (d) daily weight and frequent measurement of serum electrolytes; (e) daily intake of 100 mEq KCl; (f) spironolactone 100 mg or amiloride 10 mg/day started with reduction of KCl intake to 50 mEq/day, if after 4 days under the above regimen weight loss is less than 1 kg; (g) addition, 1 day later, of furosemide 80 mg after checking serum electrolytes; (h) doubling of daily dosage of spironolactone or amiloride if weight loss is less than 2 kg after 4 more days; and (i) increased furosemide to 120 mg if necessary. Diuretics should be stopped if flapping tremor, hypolakemia, azotemia, or alkalosis develop.

81. *Management of refractory ascites* includes several techniques: (a) plasma expansion by salt-poor albumin or by ascites ultrafiltration and reinfusion: limited by risk of infection, development of heart failure, precipitation of variceal hemorrhage, and high cost; (b) *peritoneovenous shunt*: complications are multiple, frequent, and severe—fever, leakage of peritoneal fluid, occlusion of the shunt, local and systemic infections (including bacterial endocarditis), and severe DIC (lesser degrees of DIC always occur)—reserving its use for patients in whom conservative forms of treatment have failed; and (c) portocaval anastomosis to relieve ascites: carries high mortality and the development of PSE postoperatively is common.

82. *Prognosis of patients with advanced liver disease who have ascites* is grave. Even with adequate treatment, only 40% of patients will survive 2 years after the onset of ascites. Prognosis is better when ascites have accumulated rapidly and if there is a well-defined precipitating factor (such as GI hemorrhage); prognosis is worse if liver cell failure, as evidenced by jaundice and PSE, is severe.

83. *Hepatorenal syndrome* is a functional renal failure arising either spontaneously or in response to changes in blood volume or to shifts of fluid within body compartments. The diagnosis of the syndrome rests on (a) the presence of chronic liver disease with ascites; (b) slow-onset azotemia; (c) preserved tubular function (i.e., urine to plasma osmolality ratio >1.0, urine to plasma creatinine ratio >30, urine sodium concentration <10 mEq/dl); and (d) no sustained benefit by expansion of intravascular volume. Prognosis is extremely grave.

84. *Prevention of hepatorenal syndrome* consists of (a) avoidance of diuretic overdose; (b) slow treatment of ascites; and (c) early recognition and prompt treatment of electrolyte imbalance, hemorrhage, or infection.

85. *Management of the hepatorenal syndrome* is supportive and includes restriction of fluids, sodium, potassium, and protein and withdrawal of potentially nephrotoxic drugs, such as neomycin. Renal dialysis does not improve survival.

86. *Portal blood flow* in man is about 1000–1200 ml/min. The portal vein contributes 72% of the total oxygen supply to the liver. The *normal portal pressure* is about 7 mm Hg.

87. In *cirrhosis with portal hypertension*, only 13% of the portal vein blood flow can be recovered from the hepatic veins. The remainder is drained into the systemic circulation through the following groups of collateral channels: (a) short gastric veins and the left gastric vein (coronary vein) of the portal system, which anastomose with the intercostal, diaphragmoesophageal, and azygos minor veins of the caval system at the cardia of the stomach; (b) the superior hemorrhoidal vein of the portal system, which anastomoses with the middle and inferior hemorrhoidal veins of the caval system at the anus; (c) anastomoses in the falciparum ligament through paraumbilical veins; (d) anastomoses between veins draining abdominal viscera and veins draining retroperitoneal tissues at sites where the two are in contact (e.g., liver and diaphragm, omentum, and lienorenal ligament); and (e) portal venous blood carried to the left renal vein (directly from the splenic or via diaphragmatic, pancreatic, left adrenal, or gastric veins).

88. A recent study from Yale has shown that measurement of *azygos venous blood flow* by a continuous thermal dilution technique is an index of blood flow through gastroesophageal collaterals in cirrhosis (Bosch J & Groszman RJ, Hepatology 4:424, 1984).

89. *Hepatic cirrhosis* is the most common cause of portal hypertension. *Extrahepatic portal block* may be caused by previous recurrent abdominal inflammation or by chronic pancreatitis with obstruction of the splenic vein. *Oral contraceptives* may lead to portal and hepatic venous thrombosis.

90. In *portal hypertension,* the spleen size does not correlate with portal pressure, but an enlarged spleen is the single most important diagnostic sign of portal hypertension; the diagnosis should be questioned if the spleen is of normal size.

91. *Hematemesis* is the most common presentation of portal hypertension.

92. In *portal hypertension,* varices are most often seen in the lower third of the esophagus, but they may spread upward. Esophageal varices are nearly always accompanied by gastric varices in the fundus, but the latter may be difficult to distinguish from mucosal folds on barium meal. Esophageal and gastric varices may be visualized on endoscopy as blue, rounded projections.

93. *Methods of visualizing the portal venous system* include (a) ultrasonic measurement of venous flow velocity with the pulsed Doppler flowmeter: a recently developed noninvasive technique, the results of which compare well with cineangiographic measurements; (b) percutaneous transsplenic portal venography: gives the best definition of portal venous system and estimation of portal pressure but carries the risk of intraperitoneal hemorrhage; (c) scintiphotosplenoportography: a radiotracer is injected into the spleen and serial scans are made using a gamma camera (flow patterns defined, particularly as to whether portal vein flow is hepatofugal or hepatopetal); (d) transhepatic portography: technically difficult; and (e) selective splanchnic arteriography: the hepatic arterial system is demonstrated very clearly, but the portal venous system is not and pressure cannot be measured.

94. *Wedged hepatic venous pressure (WHVP)* recorded through a catheter introduced transhepatically into an hepatic venous radicle until it can go no further represents the sinusoidal venous pressure. Pressure in the hepatic vein is measured by withdrawing the catheter about 5 cm, to the free position. Normal WHVP is 5–6 mm Hg, whereas values of about 20 mm Hg are found in patients with portal hypertension.

95. *Hepatic blood flow* can be measured by infusion of bromsulphalein (BSP) or indocyanine green and catheterization of the hepatic vein or by an analysis of the disappearance curve of indocyanine green in a peripheral artery and hepatic vein.

96. *Portal hypertension* is classified into two types: (a) *presinusoidal*: (i) *extrahepatic*: block of portal or splenic vein by infection, thrombosis, congenital anomalies, malignant tumors (of pancreas, stomach, colon, or adjacent lymph glands), acute and chronic pancreatitis, or pancreatic pseudocysts and hypercoagulable states including the use of oral contraceptives), or (ii) *intrahepatic*: the obstruction is usually in the portal tracts, e.g., schistosomiasis, congenital hepatic fibrosis, and portal zone infiltration; and (b) *sinusoidal intrahepatic*: caused by all forms of cirrhosis, as a result of distortion of the portal vascular bed and mechanical obstruction of the portal blood flow by the regenerating nodules.

97. In *presinusoidal portal hypertension*, hepatocellular function is relatively preserved; patients can better tolerate variceal hemorrhage and usually do not develop liver failure. In *intrahepatic portal hypertension*, hepatocellular disease is commonly associated, and hemorrhage frequently leads to liver failure.

98. *Idiopathic (primary) portal hypertension* has been described in which no obvious obstruction to the portal venous system can be demonstrated. This entity is common in Japan and India, but its etiology is still not established. A portal venopathy is suggested by the occlusion of intrahepatic portal radicles by portal and periportal fibrosis as well as by irregular parenchymal atrophy. A reaction to an unidentified chemical or plant toxin has been suggested.

99. *Bleeding from variceal hemorrhage* in patients with portal hypertension may follow upper respiratory infections in children and the use of nonsteroid antiinflammatory agents.

100. *Emergency endoscopy* in upper GI bleeding is indicated even in patients with documented esophageal varices, as up to 50% may bleed from other lesions, such as peptic ulcer disease, erosive gastritis, or Mallory–Weiss tears. A recent study has shown, however, that when multiple potential bleeding lesions are present and none of them is actively bleeding during endoscopy, esophageal varices are the most likely offenders; failure to prove this at endoscopy is usually attributable to delay in performing the procedure (Mitchell KJ et al, Scand J Gastroenterol 17:965, 1982).

101. The *degree of portal hypertension* correlates with the size of esophageal varices and with the chance for bleeding, but in the individual patient prediction of the chance for bleeding is inaccurate.

102. *Management of active variceal bleeding* includes (a) hospitalization with close monitoring and supportive measures (blood, plasma, vitamin K, platelets if needed, H_2-blockers because stress-induced acute mucosal ulcers are common, measures to prevent encephalopathy); (b) emergency endoscopy; (c) administration of *vasopressin*, 0.4–0.6 units/min in continuous intravenous infusion, if active variceal bleeding is seen; (d) insertion of a *Sengstaken–Blakemore* tube or one of its modifications, if bleeding continues; (e) an attempt at variceal sclerosis (see No. 103), if control of hemorrhage was achieved by one of the above measures; and (f) avoidance of emergency surgery whenever possible, but if control has not been achieved by any of the above measures a *portocaval* or *mesocaval shunt procedure* or *esophageal transection* should be done. Mortality rate is very high when shunts are done on an emergency basis. *Transhepatic variceal sclerosis* is another last-resort option in management of variceal bleeding that does not respond to a more conservative approach. Potential complications of this procedure are hemorrhage from the liver and biliary peritonitis.

103. Long-term management of variceal bleeding: (a) *Endoscopic sclerotherapy* has gained popularity in patients who have had one episode of variceal bleeding. There are only limited data from well-controlled trials to show its long-term effectiveness. A recent large study from Copenhagen supports a beneficial effect of sclerother-

apy on the incidence of rebleeding and on survival (The Copenhagen Esophageal Varices Sclerotherapy Project, N Engl J Med
311:1594, 1984). Many authorities recommend sclerotherapy as first-
line therapy for variceal bleeding. Possible complications include
disturbances in lower esophageal motility and ulcers that have the
potential to cause perforation at the injection site. Adult respiratory
distress syndrome (ARDS) and other acute and chronic pulmonary
complications have been reported but are rare. (b) *Propranolol* in a
dose that reduces the pulse rate by 25% has been shown by Lebrec
and associates to have a beneficial effect on rebleeding rates and
survival in patients with well-compensated cirrhosis (Lebrec D et
al, N Engl J Med 305:1371, 1981). Other investigators have been
unable to reproduce these results, and no effect of this medication
has been demonstrated in patients with more advanced cirrhosis.
The place of beta-blockers in the management and prevention of
variceal bleeding is still under investigation. (c) *Portosystemic shunt
surgery* to divert portal flow can reduce the incidence of rebleeding
from varices but does not improve survival. Liver failure and encephalopathy are common among patients who have undergone
portosystemic shunt surgery and the *selective distal splenorenal shunt*,
which preserves portal blood flow to the liver, seems safer in this
respect. The performance of distal splenorenal shunt requires great
surgical expertise and is associated with postoperative development of ascites.

104. Controlled trials on *prophylactic treatment of esophageal varices*
(before variceal bleeding has occurred) are being conducted, but
the effectiveness of neither prophylactic sclerotherapy nor shunt
surgery in preventing bleeding or prolonging survival in patients
with portal hypertension and varices has been demonstrated to
date.

105. *Gilbert's syndrome* affects 2–5% of the population. It is characterized by familial mild unconjugated hyperbilirubinemia, decreased plasma bilirubin clearance, and reduced hepatic UDP glu-

curonyltransferase activity. An exaggerated hyperbilirubinemia occurs after fasting and in response to administration of nicotinic acid. Liver histology and liver function tests are normal. Prognosis is excellent, with normal life expectancy.

106. *Crigler–Najjar syndrome* is characterized by a familial jaundice associated with very high serum unconjugated bilirubin levels. Deficiency of conjugating enzymes in the liver is well documented. In type I, no bilirubin-conjugating enzymes can be detected, and patients die with kernicterus during infancy. In type II, there is a deficiency in bilirubin-conjugating enzymes, but phenobarbital lowers bilirubin levels and patients survive into adulthood.

107. *Dubin–Johnson and Rotor syndromes* are characterized by familial accumulation of conjugated bilirubin in serum. Patients are mostly asymptomatic, and the condition may present as jaundice during pregnancy or after taking oral contraceptives. Defective canalicular excretion of unknown cause is thought to be the cause of the hyperbilirubinemia. The BSP test shows a diagnostic pattern—values of serum BSP after 2 hr exceed those seen after 45 min. Rotor type differs from Dubin–Johnson type in respect to pigmentation of liver (found only in Dubin–Johnson) and genetic inheritance. Both types carry an excellent prognosis.

108. *Bile acids* are metabolites of cholesterol. Synthesis is in the hepatocyte. Bile acids are secreted as glycine or taurine conjugates (3:1).

109. *Primary bile acids: cholic and chenodeoxycholic.* Intestinal flora metabolize cholic to *deoxycholic* and chenodeoxycholic to *lithocholic* acids.

110. *Lithocholic acid* is a hepatotoxin; it has a detergent effect and is minimally absorbed in the enterohepatic circulation.

111. *Bile* contains water, electrolytes, bile acids, cholesterol, phospholipids, bilirubin, and organic solutes.

112. *Total bile flow* consists of (a) bile-acid-dependent canalicular secretion (200 ml/day); (b) bile-acid-independent canalicular secretion (225 ml/day); and (c) ductular secretion (180 ml/day).

113. *Secretin, CCK,* and *gastrin* stimulate bile flow.

114. The concentration of *bile in the duodenum* is 5–10 mM in the basal state and 13–46 mM after contraction of the gallbladder.

115. *Bile salt pool*: 5–10 mM (1–4 g). *Enterohepatic circulation*: 3–12 times daily.

116. *Cholestasis* involves impaired bile formation. The lack of carrier for bilirubin excretion causes hyperbilirubinemia.

117. *Important histological characteristics of cholestasis* include (a) accumulation of bile in centrizonal areas, Kupffer cells, and canaliculi; (b) feathery degeneration of centrizonal hepatocytes; and (c) late portal zone fibrosis.

118. *Xanthomata* will develop in prolonged cholestasis, mainly when serum total lipids exceed 1800 mg/dl or serum cholesterol exceeds 450 mg/dl for more than 3 months.

119. *Osteomalacia* from failure to absorb calcium and vitamin D in chronic cholestasis will not manifest earlier than 2 years after the onset of cholestasis and cannot be predicted from serum calcium and phosphate levels.

120. *Copper* accumulates in the liver in cholestasis.

121. *Portal hypertension* and *hepatocellular failure* in cholestasis develop later than in other processes leading to cirrhosis.

122. *Management of chronic cholestasis* includes less than 40 g dietary fat; medium-chain triglycerides (MCT); vitamins A, D, and K; calcium; cholestyramine; and phenobarbital.

123. *Cholestyramine* is effective only in partial biliary obstruction, should be administered before meals, and relieves pruritus within 4–7 days.

124. *Cholestasis* (even severe) is not a contraindication for liver biopsy as long as PT is not over 3 sec off control after vitamin K and as long as platelets are over 80,000/mm^3.

125. *Hepatic bile* contains Na 150 mEq/liter, K 4 mEq/liter, Cl 95 mEq/liter, HCO$_3$ 10 mEq/liter. Thus, in external biliary fistula, the primary loss is of Na and K.

126. *Hepatic histology in extrahepatic cholestasis* is characterized by (a) multiple tortuous bile ducts in the portal zone; (b) polymorphonuclear leukocytes around bile ducts if ascending cholangitis is caused by the obstruction; (c) focal necrosis of heptocytes starting in the middle of the lobe and spreading to the portal triads; (d) "bile lakes" (ruptured interlobular bile ducts); and (e) portal fibrosis as a late result.

127. *Hepatic histology in intrahepatic cholestasis* is different from histology in extrahepatic cholestasis; cholangitis is absent, bile ducts within the liver are not dilated, and bile duct multiplication and biliary necrosis are not seen.

128. *Intrahepatic cholestasis* may be classified according to the site of involvement on the biliary tree: (a) *hepatocellular*: viral hepatitis, alcoholic hepatitis, postnecrotic cirrhosis, drugs, and Dubin–Johnson–Rotor; (b) *canalicular*: sex hormones and pregnancy; and (c) *biliary*: chlorpromazine, benign recurrent cholestasis, primary biliary cirrhosis, biliary atresia, sclerosing cholangitis, and cholangiocarcinoma.

129. *Primary biliary cirrhosis (PBC)* (a) is a chronic inflammatory disease involving the small interlobular bile ducts that progresses to cirrhosis and may lead to liver failure and/or portal hypertension; (b) has an unknown etiology, but there seems to be familial clustering and there is an increase in the incidence of serological antibodies in healthy relatives of patients; (c) may be tested with *antimitochondrial antibodies* as the best immunological marker, being positive in 90% of patients, but they are not specific and may be found in patients with chronic active or drug-induced hepatitis; (d) has clinical features including 90% incidence in females, usually between the ages of 40 and 59, presenting with pruritus; jaundice may be concomitant or follows a few months to years after the onset of pruritus, pigmentation, steatorrhea, and skin xanthomas; severe bone changes occur when jaundice is deep; (e) has a variable course—patients may be asymptomatic, and survival for this group has recently been reported to be no different from that in a control population for at least 12 years after diagnosis; the average length of survival from the onset of symptoms in symptomatic patients is about 12 years; (f) is commonly associated with extrahepatic diseases, including systemic lupus erythematosus (SLE), scleroderma (with or without Sjogren's syndrome), rheumatoid arthritis, dermatomyositis, celiac disease, and membranous glomerulonephritis; cholelithiasis has been reported in about 40% of cases; (g) exhibits biochemical findings including increased levels of serum bilirubin, alkaline phosphatase, and IgM; (h) displays histological findings that may be divided into four stages: stage 1 (damaged bile ducts surrounded by an infiltrate of lymphocytes, epithelioid cells, and plasma cells, and granulomas may be present), stage 2 (ductular proliferation, fibrosis, acute and chronic inflammatory infiltration, and lymphoid aggregates, and Mallory hyaline may be seen in liver cells), stage 3 (scarring with acellular septa extending from the portal tracts), and stage 4 (cirrhosis); (i) carries a better prognosis in association with portal fibrosis limited to the portal triad, onset at young age, normal-size liver, and normal serum bilirubin; and (j) is treated symptomatically as for other chronic cholestatic states; steroids are contraindicated due to increased bone damage, and other immunosuppressive agents as well as D-penicillamine did not improve liver function tests or prognosis. Primary biliary cirrhosis has been considered by many authorities to be one of the prime indications for liver transplantation.

130. *Primary sclerosing cholangitis* (a) is a chronic fibrosing inflammatory process involving all parts of the biliary tract; (b) shows the walls of the bile ducts (extrahepatic and intrahepatic) and gall-bladder to be infiltrated with lymphocytes, plasma cells, and eo-sinophils with fibrosis; (c) in about 75% of cases is associated with *ulcerative colitis*, which preceded sclerosing cholangitis; (d) is associated with Riedel's struma, pancreatitis, retroperitoneal fibrosis, immune-deficiency syndromes, and rarely cholangiocarcinoma; (e) has clinical features including male-to-female ratio of 2:1 and a common presentation with jaundice, pruritus, weight loss, RUQ pain, and acute cholangitis, with possible manifestations of portal hypertension, and occasional lack of symptomatology; (f) is detected by the preferred diagnostic technique of ERCP, which shows irregular stricturing and dilatation (beading) of the intrahepatic and extrahepatic bile ducts; (g) has complications including recurrent cholangitis and portal hypertension; (h) has a mean survival from onset of symptoms of about 7 years, but patients can remain asymptomatic for many years; (i) shows a disappointing response to treatment, which includes surgery in complete main duct obstruction and, for removal of stones, endoprostheses when strictures are not amenable to surgical correction and antimicrobial agents for episodes of acute cholangitis; removal of diseased colon does not affect the course of biliary tract disease; and (j) has been surgically treated with liver transplantation, performed successfully.

131. The basic histological picture of *acute viral hepatitis* (A, B, or NANB) includes (a) hepatic cell necrosis, which is more prominent in the center of the lobules, and cellular infiltration, which is more prominent in the portal tracts; (b) hyperplasia of Kupffer cells, neutrophils, and eosinophils; (c) acidophilic bodies; (d) centrizonal cholestasis; and (e) commonly bile duct proliferation.

132. *Aplastic anemia* may occur in all three forms of hepatitis.

133. *The three types of viral hepatitis*—A, B, and NANB—run essentially the same clinical course, but type B tends to be more severe.

134. In *viral hepatitis,* the prodromal period lasts a few days to 3 weeks and consists of anorexia, nausea, abdominal pain, fever, loss of desire to smoke or to drink alcohol, malaise, and fatigue. Headache may be severe, but this is uncommon.

135. A *cholestatic variant of viral hepatitis* occurs and should be differentiated from extrahepatic obstruction by the acute onset of the latter.

136. In *fulminant hepatitis,* clinical deterioration develops rapidly and mortality rate is high. Repeated vomiting, fetor hepaticus, confusion, and drowsiness are grave prognostic signs. The clinical and laboratory features are those of acute liver failure (see No. 72). Prognosis is unrelated to bilirubin and enzyme levels, but PT correlates with prognosis. Survival is about 33% in fulminant hepatitis caused by hepatitis B virus (HBV) and 13% for fulminant-type NANB.

137. In *hepatitis A* (a) the cause is an RNA virus, a picornavirus in the genus *Enterovirus;* (b) the virus is excreted in the stool from about 2 weeks before until 1 week after the onset of jaundice; (c) serum IgM antibody to hepatitis A virus (HAV) is indicative of a recent infection, persisting in the serum for 2–6 months, while IgG anti-HAV is detectable for many years and probably confers immunity for life; (d) chronic carriers have not been identified; (e) rapid progress is being made for production of attenuated live vaccine but it is still unavailable; (f) in urban areas, most of the adult population (60–70%) show circulating anti-HAV; and (g) the course is usually clinically mild, frequently unicteric, and rarely fulminant. Long-term prognosis is excellent.

138. In *hepatitis B* (a) the cause is a DNA virus, the virion of which is composed of a core containing DNA polymerase, double-stranded DNA, core antigen (HBcAg), an e antigen (HBeAg), and a surface consisting of a surface antigen (HBsAg); (b) HBsAg appears in the blood about 6 weeks after infection and disappears by 3 months;

in early acute hepatitis (when HBsAg is still not demonstrable), diagnosis can be proved by IgM anti-HBc (mainly the 19 S IgM antibody, while the 7 S IgM antibody indicates a chronic disease); (c) persistence of HBsAg for more than 6 months implies a carrier state; anti-HBs appears about 3 months after the onset of illness and appears to confer immunity; 10–15% of patients with acute hepatitis B never develop anti-HBs; (d) HBeAg appears after about 1 week of illness and usually disappears by 2 weeks; persistence implies ongoing disease; the appearance of anti-HBe follows the disappearance of HBeAg and it is present for many months; (e) IgG anti-HBc appears early in the course and persists for many months; (f) HBeAg and DNA polymerase imply ongoing infectivity; and (g) in carriers and in chronic hepatitis B, hepatocytes may be stained orange with orcein.

139. In *hepatitis B* (a) spread is largely by whole blood and its products; health personnel and homosexuals are at high risk; (b) the carrier rate of HBsAg varies from 0.1 to 0.2% in Western developed countries to 15% in certain areas of the Far East; (c) subclinical episodes are common; (d) clinical features are similar to those of hepatitis A but tend to be more severe; and (e) serum-sickness-like syndrome may be part of the prodrome and includes fever, urticaria, and arthropathy of small joints.

140. *Endoscopy does not cause transmission of hepatitis B*, as shown by several studies.

141. In *hepatitis B* (a) a carrier state occurs in about 10% of patients suffering from acute hepatitis B and is manifested by persistence of HBsAg for more than 6 months; (b) carriers seldom revert to a negative HBsAg state, but conversion may occur after many years; (c) the extent of infectivity of a carrier has not been established but is probably small; (d) histological changes on liver biopsy are common even in carriers of HBsAg who appear to be healthy; (e) positive serum HBeAg or IgM anti-HBc indicates infectivity due to ongoing disease; (f) the likelihood of a persistent HBsAg carrier state is greater if hepatitis B occurs before 3 years of age than if it is acquired later in childhood; and (g) a recent 10-year prospective cohort study of carriers over 40 years of age confirmed the high risk of hepatocellular carcinoma in these patients (Beasley RP et al, Lancet 2:1129, 1981) (see No. 212).

142. *Conditions associated with circulating immune complexes containing HBsAg* include (a) polyarteritis; (b) glomerulonephritis (a rare association exists between membranous or membranoproliferative glomerulonephritis and chronic hepatitis B infection); and (c) essential mixed cryoglobulinemia (the exact relationship with hepatitis B has not been determined).

143. *NANB hepatitis* (a) probably accounts for about 75% of post-transfusion hepatitis and 15–20% of sporadic hepatitis; (b) still awaits a suitable diagnostic test or a serological marker; (c) is largely blood spread; (d) has an average incubation period of 7 weeks, with clinical and laboratory features similar to those of hepatitis A or B, but serum enzyme levels tend to wax and wane for months; (e) is uncommonly associated with fulminant hepatitis; (f) commonly leads to the development of chronic hepatitis, in about 25% of cases, is usually mild, and improves with time, but cirrhosis may ensue.

144. *Delta agent:* (a) The agent is a defective RNA virus that requires the helper function of HBV for its multiplication; (b) it has been shown to be present in epidemics of acute hepatitis B in areas with a high HBV carrier rate, and the delta marker rate was recently found to be 34% in fulminant hepatitis in Los Angeles (Govindarajan S et al, Gastroenterology 86:1417, 1984); (c) it is common among drug addicts; (d) it causes a particularly progressive chronic hepatitis (now called hepatitis D) and is usually but not necessarily HBeAg negative; and (d) a sensitive enzyme immunoassay for D Ag and anti-D has recently been developed.

145. *Prevention and treatment of viral hepatitis* include (a) immune globulin, 0.02 ml/kg body weight IM within 2 weeks after exposure, to modify hepatitis A infection to a subclinical form, indicated for household contacts of an index case; (b) passive immunization with hepatitis B immune globulin, indicated in the neonate of the HBsAg-positive mother (0.5 ml at birth and at 3 and 6 months), for sexual contacts of a patient with acute hepatitis B (3–5 ml and repeated after 1 month), and for accidental needle stick or mucous membrane exposure (same dose as for sexual contacts); (c) active immunization with the HBsAg vaccine, indicated postexposure for the three groups mentioned in (b) and as prophylaxis for health-care workers, hemodialysis patients, and other immunosuppressed persons (a second dose is given at 1 month and a third at 6 months) (the efficacy of passive immunization with immune globulin to prevent NANB hepatitis has not been determined and active immunization is still unavailable); (d) general measures such as a high-calorie fluid-rich diet, intravenous fluids if nausea and vomiting are severe, avoidance of tranquilizers, alcohol, and any medications that are not essential, and restriction of strenuous physical activity; corticosteroids should not be used; enteric precautions seem appropriate for hepatitis A and blood precautions for hepatitis B and NANB; and (e) follow-up evaluation of patients until resolution of abnormalities in liver function tests.

146. In *fulminant hepatitis,* no treatment is known to speed resolution or to increase survival rate, but emphasis should be given to vigorous maintenance of vital functions and prompt recognition and treatment of life-threatening complications. Such measures include close monitoring of vital signs, serum electrolytes, creatinine, glucose, and coagulation profile. Encephalopathy is common and should be treated promptly; the same is true for fluid and electrolyte imbalance, respiratory failure, cerebral edema, and GI bleeding from erosive gastritis. Artificial hepatic support devices are still under development, but successful liver transplantation has been reported in a few patients (see No. 218).

147. In *hepatitis B*, a general rule is that the more severe the acute attack, the less likely the chronic sequelae. Patients who survive an attack of fulminant hepatitis usually recover completely without the development of chronic disease.

148. *Chronic hepatitis* is a chronic inflammatory reaction in the liver that does not improve for at least 6 months. It is divided into three types: (a) *chronic persistent hepatitis (CPH)*: the mononuclear infiltrate and fibrosis expand the portal zone, but the limiting plate is intact, and piecemeal necrosis is not seen (CPH does not progress to cirrhosis); (b) *chronic lobular hepatitis*: histological features are similar to changes in acute viral hepatitis (intralobular inflammation and necrosis but no piecemeal or bridging necrosis), but duration is longer than 3 months (chronic lobular hepatitis does not progress to cirrhosis); and (c) *chronic active hepatitis (CAH)*: the inflammatory infiltrate expands the portal areas and extends into the lobules, eroding the limiting plate and leading to piecemeal necrosis; in its severe form, CAH often progresses to cirrhosis; bridging necrosis (portal–central or portal–portal) is considered prognostically significant in predicting the progression of CAH to cirrhosis.

149. *Chronic persistent hepatitis (CPH)* (a) may follow viral hepatitis B, NANB, and alcoholic hepatitis or complicate long-standing inflammatory bowel disease; (b) is asymptomatic in most patients but some patients may complain of mild fatigue and anorexia; physical examination is normal; (c) may show slightly to moderately disturbed liver function tests; (d) is treated with reassurance—steroids or immunosuppressive agents should not be given, and no dietary limitations are indicated; and (e) carries a favorable prognosis and no progression to cirrhosis occurs.

150. *Chronic lobular hepatitis* (a) is rare; (b) is characterized by a course of remissions and relapses marked by elevated transaminases; (c) may display positive anti-smooth-muscle antibodies and antimitochondrial antibodies; and (d) carries a favorable prognosis;

clinical or biochemical exacerbations respond to corticosteroids; cirrhosis does not develop.

151. *Chronic active hepatitis* has the following characteristics: (a) It may follow viral hepatitis B, NANB, or other viral infections such as rubella or cytomegalovirus or may represent the hepatic involvement of alpha$_1$-antitrypsin deficiency, alcoholic liver disease, drug-induced liver damage, and Wilson's disease. Another form of CAH is the autoimmune type, also called "lupoid" hepatitis or idiopathic CAH. (b) CAH that follows hepatitis B is more common in males, serum HBsAg is present, associated autoimmune disorders are rare, serum gammaglobulins may increase moderately, the presence of smooth muscle antibodies or LE cells is rare, and the risk of the development of primary liver cancer is high. Clinical presentation is variable: patients may be asymptomatic with only biochemical evidence of activity or may present with jaundice or signs of portal hypertension. Response to corticosteroids is unpredictable, and a few studies have shown that steroid therapy in HBsAg-positive CAH may increase mortality. Most authorities recommend a therapeutic trial with prednisolone, 20 mg/day, in symptomatic patients demonstrating "histological activity" (bridging necrosis or multilobular necrosis). If after 6 months of therapy there is no clinical, biochemical, or histological improvement, the drug should be discontinued. Antiviral therapy with interferon and adenine arabinoside (ara-a) or immunostimulation with transfer factor and levamisol have not proved efficacious. (c) CAH commonly follows posttransfusion NANB hepatitis and is characterized by waxing and waning of clinical and laboratory features. The rate of progression to cirrhosis is unknown and, as for CAH of hepatitis B, corticosteroids have not proved of great benefit and an effective specific therapy has not been established. (d) CAH of the autoimmune type ("lupoid") is more common in women under 30 years of age (with a female to male ratio of 3:1); HBsAg is absent in the serum, elevated IgG levels are common, smooth muscle antibody is detected in the blood of about 70% of patients; antinuclear antibodies, rheumatoid factor, and LE cells may also be present. Association with other autoimmune disorders such as thyroiditis, glomerulonephritis, pernicious anemia, Coombs-positive hemolytic anemia, and Sjögren syndrome may occur. The risk of the development of primary liver cancer is low, and response to corticosteroid therapy is good (40 mg prednisolone should be given daily with gradual tapering to maintenance dose of 15–20 mg over 4–6 weeks). After 6 months, clinical and biochemical evidence of activity disappears in a large percentage of patients, and steroids can be discontinued. When relapse occurs, reinstitution of the same regimen usually suppresses activity of the disease. The overwhelming majority of patients progress to cirrhosis.

152. *Drug-induced liver disease*: (a) Drugs can induce an acute or chronic disease of the liver. Acute injury may lead to *necrosis, steatosis,* or *cholestasis*. Chronic injury may be manifested in the form of *chronic active hepatitis, fatty liver, phospholipidosis, vascular lesion, granulomas, cholestasis, cirrhosis, portal hypertension,* or *neoplasms*. (b) Mechanisms of drug hepatotoxicity include (i) a direct action on the liver cell (rare); (ii) combination of a metabolic product of the drug with essential cell proteins, causing necrosis (after exhaustion of glutathione stores), a dose-dependent reaction with a microscopic appearance characterized by centrizonal necrosis, fatty change, some inflammatory reaction, and periportal fibrosis (acetaminophen toxicity is an example); and (iii) an immunological reaction that is not dose dependent; only a small percentage of those receiving the drug are affected; diagnosis can be proved by rechallenge, which is not always ethically justified (halothane hepatotoxicity is an example).

153. In *acetaminophen (paracetamol) hepatotoxicity*, (a) doses over 10–15 g lead to hepatic necrosis that becomes overt after 24–48 hr; (b) myocardial and renal damage and hypoglycemia may be prominent; (c) serum transaminase levels and PT are excessively increased; (d) if 4 hr after ingestion blood levels exceed 300 μg/ml there is 100% incidence of hepatic toxicity; if after 12 hr level is less than 50 μg/ml prognosis is good; (e) treatment includes *N-acetyl-cysteine (Mucomist)*, 140 mg/kg PO, followed by 70 mg/kg at 4-hr intervals for 72 hr; if the IV route is used, 150 mg/kg should be administered in 200 ml dextrose in 5% water over a 15-min period, followed by 50 mg/kg over the next 4 hr, 100 mg/kg over the next 16 hr; (f) patients arriving after more than 24 hr who have toxic blood levels should be managed as for fulminant hepatic failure, since *N*-acetylcysteine will be of no use; and (g) *charcoal column hemoperfusion* may be helpful when hepatic failure develops.

154. *Carbontetrachloride (CCl₄)* and other chlorinated hydrocarbons (e.g., trichlorethylene) may induce hepatic necrosis, acute renal failure (ARF), and drowsiness. Acute poisoning should be treated with a high-calorie, high-carbohydrate diet, the usual regimen for hepatic failure and hemodialysis when renal failure ensues.

155. *Methotrexate* is commonly used in the treatment of psoriasis. Prolonged therapy may result in hepatic fibrosis and subsequently cirrhosis. Liver cell carcinoma can develop. Periodic liver biopsies in patients on long-term methotrexate therapy should be done to detect fibrosis at an early stage.

156. *Azathioprine (Imuran)* may lead to *cholestasis, venoocclusive disease*, or *peliosis hepatis*.

157. *Cyclosporin A*, which is commonly given to patients undergoing liver or kidney transplants, has been reported to induce raised transaminase levels, but it generally does not result in clinical illness.

158. *Salicylates* and other *nonsteroidal antiinflammatory drugs* can all cause liver damage, usually of a mixed cholestatic–hepatitic type. Both acute hepatic injury and chronic active hepatitis have been reported.

159. *Amiodarone*, an antiarrhythmic agent with an unusually long half-life, may produce features of alcoholic liver disease including Mallory bodies, as well as phospholipidotic small droplets.

160. *Isoniazid* can lead to transient elevation of SGOT in about 20% of patients. Alcohol consumption and advanced age are associated with increased risk. Rapid acetylators are at increased risk of developing liver damage, and combination with an enzyme inducer such as rifampicin further increases the risk and may even lead to fulminant hepatitis. In most cases, SGOT levels are transiently elevated with no resulting symptoms and with subsidance despite continued therapy, but when elevation is prolonged and medication is not stopped, hepatitis with jaundice may ensue. The hepatitis usually resolves on stopping the drug, but continued administration may lead to CAH and even *cirrhosis*.

161. *Methyldopa* may lead to asymptomatic elevation of serum transaminase in 5% of users. It usually subsides despite continued drug administration, but more severe liver damage with bridging and multilobular necrosis has been reported to occur uncommonly.

162. *Halothane* hepatotoxicity occurs in about 1/10,000 anesthesias in adults; it is very rare in children. A specific halothane-related antibody has been found, indicating sensitization to halothane-altered liver cell membrane components. Fever occurs about 7 days after exposure and jaundice appears 2–3 days later, but hepatitis is more common after multiple exposure; obese elderly female patients seem particularly at risk. Early onset of jaundice is a grave prognostic sign. In one large series, mortality was 46%, but in those who recover, chronic liver disease does not develop.

163. *Chlorpromazine* causes cholestatic jaundice in 1–2% of patients. The reaction is not dose dependent and usually occurs during the first 4 weeks. Pruritus may precede the cholestatic jaundice, and complete recovery is the rule if the drug is discontinued, although prolonged cholestatic jaundice with steatorrhea is occasionally seen.

164. *Oral contraceptives* may affect the hepatobiliary system in various ways: (a) cholestatic jaundice may appear during one of the first three cycles of administration, a rare complication; centrizonal necrosis is seen on biopsy, and prognosis is excellent if the medication is discontinued; (b) women on longterm oral contraceptives have a twofold increase in incidence of gallstones over incidence in controls; (c) the Budd–Chiari syndrome is associated with the use of oral contraceptives of the estrogen–progesterone type; and (d) a rare association of oral contraceptives with *hepatic adenomas, focal nodular hyperplasia,* and *peliosis hepatis* is well documented; very rarely, an association with *hepatocellular carcinoma* and with *cholangiocarcinoma* has been reported.

165. *Postoperative jaundice* may occur as a result of (a) bilirubin load from blood transfusions; (b) hepatic hypoperfusion caused by anesthetics and/or shock; or (c) halothane and other hepatotoxic drugs used for induction of anesthesia. A cholestatic jaundice of unknown mechanism may occur on the first or second postoperative day, reaching its height between the fourth and tenth days, and disappearing within approximately 15 days.

166. In *acute heart failure* or *shock*, congested central areas with local hemorrhage are seen on light microscopy. If shock is prolonged (longer than 24 hr), hepatic necrosis may occur.

167. In the *Budd–Chiari syndrome* (a) the cause is obstruction of hepatic veins at any site from the efferent vein of the lobule to the entry of the inferior vena cava into the right atrium; (b) etiological factors include intrahepatic venoocclusive disease (e.g., azathioprine-induced liver damage, acute alcoholic hepatitis), congenital webs, tumors occluding the hepatic vein or inferior vena cava, oral contraceptives, constrictive pericarditis, and hypercoagulable states such as polycythemia; (c) clinical features include hepatomegaly, abdominal pain, and ascites; (d) hepatic histology shows centrizonal sinusoidal distention and pooling; (e) the most frequent complications are thrombosis of the portal vein and pulmonary embolism; and (f) treatment consists of controlling ascites by conservative measures, taking care of the etiological factor where possible (e.g., resection of webs, venesection in polycythemia) and side-to-side portocaval shunt if the portal vein and inferior vena cava are patent, or mesoatrial shunt if the inferior vena cava is obstructed; anticoagulants or fibrinolysins are of no benefit.

168. *Hepatic cirrhosis* is a diffuse process with fibrosis and nodule formation. It is the common end result of many liver diseases. The most common causes in Western countries are viral hepatitis, alcohol, and chronic active hepatitis. In about 25% of patients, the etiology is unknown and the term used is *cryptogenic cirrhosis.* Cirrhosis may result in *hepatocellular failure,* with jaundice, encephalopathy, hypoalbuminemia, ascites, high transaminase levels, and prothrombin deficiency, and/or in *portal hypertension,* with splenomegaly, esophageal varices, and ascites.

169. *Liver cirrhosis* may be associated with (a) esophageal and gastric varices and PUD; (b) splenomegaly and abdominal wall venous collaterals; (c) steatorrhea (due to chronic pancreatitis of alcoholism or reduced bile salt secretion); (d) abdominal hernia (due to ascites); (e) primary liver cancer (except in biliary and cardiac cirrhosis); (f) gallstones (mainly pigment stones); (g) digital clubbing (mainly in biliary cirrhosis); (h) Dupuytrens' contracture (mainly in alcoholic cirrhosis); (i) infection (frequent septicemia, spontaneous bacterial peritonitis); and (j) a continuous low-grade fever in one-third of patients with active advanced cirrhosis; it is more common in alcoholics.

170. In *hepatic cirrhosis,* elevation of serum globulin is common, mainly gamma-globulin (failure of the sick liver to clear intestinal antigens?).

171. In *hepatic cirrhosis,* needle biopsy should always be done unless a coagulation defect or significant ascites are present. The histological appearance may give a clue to etiology and activity, and serial biopsies help assess progression. A sampling error is common due to the tendency of the commonly used needles to aspirate the soft parenchyma and leave fibrous tissue behind.

172. *Prognosis in hepatic cirrhosis* (a) depends on etiology (alcoholics who abstain do better than "cryptogenic" cirrhotics); (b) is improved when a precipitating factor of decompensation can be identified (e.g., hemorrhage, infection); (c) is poor when there are signs of jaundice, ascites, encephalopathy developing in the course of hepatocellular failure, hypoalbuminemia (<2.5 g/dl), hyponatremia unrelated to diuretic therapy, and persistent hypoprothrombinemia; and (d) is not correlated with serum transaminase and globulin levels.

173. *The management of hepatic cirrhosis* consists of a well-balanced diet (no limitation in fat consumption is necessary) in well-compensated cirrhosis, early detection of signs indicating hepatocellular failure, and treatment of complications of the latter (ascites, encephalopathy, portal hypertension). Therapeutic modalities aimed at preventing collagen synthesis or progressive fibrosis are still unavailable.

174. *Alcoholic liver disease* is related to the amount of alcohol consumed. Most alcoholics with cirrhosis have consumed about 190 g alcohol daily for 10 years, but individual variations exist. A "safe" limit may be the consumption of not more than 60 g alcohol daily for men and 20 g for women. There may be a genetic predisposition for liver damage from alcohol, as only 25% of alcoholics show severe liver damage and 50% show milder damage.

175. *The pathogenesis of alcoholic liver injury* invovles (a) stimulation of fibrogenesis and collagen synthesis; (b)immunological stimulation leading to progressive destruction of liver cells (hyaline may be the antigen); (c) increased hepatic oxygen consumption, with centrizonal areas the last to receive oxygen, and these regions suffer most; and (d) decreased consumption of dietary protein leading to decreased capacity of the liver to metabolize alcohol and to synthesize the lipoprotein necessary for transport of fat from the liver.

176. *The histopathology of alcoholic liver disease* is characterized by (a) fatty infiltration; (b) Mallory hyaline (particularly in centrizonal areas); (c) Kupffer cell proliferation; (d) cholestasis; (e) polymorphs surrounding necrotic cells characteristic of the "acute" phase; (f) in very advanced stages, a shrinking liver, disappearance of the fatty infiltration, and development of a fibrotic process (perivenular and perisinusoidal) leading to micronodular cirrhosis; and (g) mega-mitochondria seen on electron microscopy.

177. *A histological picture similar to alcoholic liver disease* may be seen in *severe obesity, Wilson's disease, diabetes mellitus, after jejunoileal bypass,* and in *Indian childhood cirrhosis.*

178. *Delirium tremens (DT)* can be differentiated from hepatic precoma by the following features: (a) in DT, patients are alert and hyperactive while in hepatic precoma drowsiness is the rule; and (b) the tremor is fine in DT and flapping in hepatic precoma.

179. *Alcoholic cirrhosis* is not always preceded by episodes of acute alcoholic hepatitis. It may present as any end-stage liver disease, and only the history of alcohol abuse suggests the diagnosis.

180. In *alcoholic cirrhosis,* portal hypertension may be caused by (a) regeneration nodules; (b) pressure exerted on portal venous drainage by fatty infiltration; and (c) sclerosing hyaline necrosis which may add a postsinusoidal component.

181. *Prognosis of patients with established alcoholic cirrhosis* depends on the presence of portal hypertension and on drinking habits. Before the onset of portal hypertension, survival may be significantly improved by abstinence.

182. *Mortality rate in acute alcoholic hepatitis* is 2–8%. Prolonged PT (especially if unresponsive to vitamin K), severe hyperbilirubinemia, and hypoalbuminemia are poor prognostic signs.

183. *Liver biopsy* is indicated in patients with alcoholic liver disease when abnormal liver function tests persist for 3–6 months, as, according to recent studies, *perivenular fibrosis* at the fatty liver stage is an early sign of impending cirrhosis. These changes are still reversible in most cases, provided strict abstinence from alcohol is practiced.

184. *Treatment of acute alcoholic hepatitis* includes (a) complete alcohol withdrawal; (b) high-calorie diet—sometimes anorexia is severe and parenteral alimentation is needed, including daily infusion of 70–90 g amino acids (a mixture rich in BCAAs and poor in aromatic amino acids is advocated to minimize the risk of encephalopathy); (c) steroids—as a last-resort option in severe unresponsive cases although they are not recommended on a routine basis and may even have deleterious effects; and (d) propylthiouracil, colchicine, D-penicillamine, and the infusion of glucagon and insulin, which have been reported in a few studies to have a beneficial effect, but further studies are needed to confirm these initial observations.

185. Despite *vitamin A deficiency* in chronic liver disease, excess intake of this vitamin has been reported to cause *hepatic fibrosis* with *portal hypertension*. In replenishment of vitamin A, it is recommended that the daily dose not exceed 2000 IU.

186. Excess *iron* deposits in hepatocytes may lead to cellular damage resulting in the development of cirrhosis. Ferritin, hemosiderin, and lipofuscin may be found in the liver when iron overload occurs.

187. In *idiopathic hemochromatosis*, (a) the etiology is a rare genetically determined (autosomal recessive) metabolic disorder with increased iron absorption over many years; (b) portal zone fibrosis in hemochromatosis may develop into macronodular cirrhosis; fibrosis of the pancreas is common, and the spleen, heart, and intestine are also involved; (c) common manifestations include arthritis (67% of patients, involves metacarpophalangeal joints, knees, and hips, and chondrocalcinosis is seen in articular cartilage), bronze skin pigmentation, hepatosplenomegaly, weakness, loss of libido, testicular atrophy, loss of body hair, diabetes mellitus, and cardio-myopathy with dysrhythmia; (d) diagnosis is made by liver biopsy showing increased iron stores in hepatocytes and Kupffer cells and varying degrees of hepatic fibrosis or cirrhosis; liver CT scan may help assess liver iron stores; serum ferritin and transferrin saturation are the best screening tests but patients with early disease may have normal values; (e) HLA types A3, B7, and B14 are particularly common when compared with the general population, and screening of relatives should be done as relatives homozygous with the proband are at high risk of developing the disease; (e) treatment consists of frequent phlebotomies; as body iron stores in these patients may be increased up to 100 – fold over normal, some patients require weekly or biweekly phlebotomies for 1–2 years; Hct levels should be followed and serum ferritin, iron saturation, reticulocyte count, and RBC indices are helpful in assessing whether an iron – deficient state has been reached; and (f) the above treatment improves liver function tests and probably prolongs survival, but about 15% of patients show the development of *hepatocellular carcinoma*, and its incidence is not reduced by therapy.

188. In *beta-(homozygous) thalassemia*, increased iron stores result from frequent blood transfusion and iron absorption rates disproportionate to the body stores. Treatment consists of low-iron diet and chelation therapy with desferrioxamine. Hepatic fibrosis may be impeded by this therapy.

189. In *cirrhosis*, especially *alcoholic cirrhosis*, increased hepatic iron stores result from increased iron absorption and the high iron content of wine. A distinction from idiopathic hemochromatosis is made on the basis of family history and liver biopsy. Treatment should be of the primary disorder, as removal of iron has not been found to improve morbidity or survival.

190. In *Wilson's disease* (a) the etiology is an inherited (autosomal recessive) disease characterized by cirrhosis of the liver, degeneration of basal ganglia in the brain, a pigmented ring in the periphery of the cornea (Kayser–Fleischer ring), and renal tubular lesions; (b) increased copper deposition is considered responsible for the lesions; (c) symptoms commonly appear in childhood or in youth; (d) liver histology is variable and may show *periportal fibrosis*, an *alcoholic-hepatitis-like picture* or *macronodular cirrhosis*; cirrhosis in the young should always arouse suspicion of Wilson's disease; (e) clinical presentation is also variable and includes fulminant hepatitis, chronic active hepatitis, cirrhosis with portal hypertension, and neurological symptoms (the latter are more common in patients presenting after age 20); (f) the diagnosis is made by demonstrating corneal Kayser–Fleischer rings, hepatic copper concentration of more than 250 μg/g dry tissue, and urinary copper of more than 100 μg/24 hr; serum ceruloplasmin is usually below 20 mg/dl; (g) treatment consists of D-penicillamine (should be given even to asymptomatic patients), 250 mg qid (adult dose) before meals; the dose should be increased to 2–3 g/day if improvement is not observed within 3–6 months; pyridoxine, 25 mg/day, should be supplemented; response to treatment is manifested by the disappearance of the corneal rings and by improvement in neurological symptoms; the liver disease may beocme inactive with improvement in liver function; (h) few reports on successful *liver transplantation* in patients with advanced liver failure caused by Wilson's disease have been published; and (i) prognosis is good when treatment is started early in the course, before the onset of neurological symptoms or advanced liver disease; acute neurological symptoms, dystonia, and early acute liver failure carry a poor prognosis.

191. In *obese patients*, fatty infiltration of the liver is common, but the fatty changes do not lead to cirrhosis.

192. *Total parenteral nutrition (TPN)* may be complicated by cholestasis. In infants, prolonged TPN has been reported to result in liver failure.

193. In *diabetes mellitus*, hepatomegaly with increased glycogen contents occurs uncommonly in patients with the insulin-sensitive type, mainly in uncontrolled patients and in diabetic ketoacidosis. Fatty liver, probably related to obesity, may be seen in patients with insulin-insensitive diabetes.

194. In *alpha$_1$-antitrypsin deficiency* (a) the etiology is an inherited disorder with decreased serum alpha$_1$-antitrypsin levels; (b) the alpha$_1$-globulin is an inhibitor of trypsin and other proteases *in vitro* that may have a protective function in various tissues; (c) clinical features include hepatitic–cholestatic jaundice during the neonatal period, cirrhosis in childhood or early adulthood, and pulmonary emphysema; pulmonary and hepatic disease rarely occur in the same patient; (d) diagnosis should be suspected with neonatal jaundice and confirmed by low or absent serum alpha$_1$-antitrypsin. Methods for prenatal diagnosis of homozygotes have been recently developed; and (e) there is no specific treatment, although *liver transplantation* has been performed successfully in a few patients to date.

195. Proliferation of *giant cells* is the common reaction of the neonatal liver to various insults. It may be induced by viruses (HBV, CMV, herpes, rubella, coxsackie), bacteria, metabolic disorders (e.g., alpha$_1$-antitrypsin deficiency, galactosemia), TPN, or biliary atresia, or may be "idiopathic."

196. *Viral hepatitis in the neonatal period* leads to a high incidence of chronic hepatitis and cirrhosis.

197. *Hepatitis B* may be transmitted from an HBeAg-positive mother (or rarely, from a mother who is an asymptomatic carrier) to the newborn through breast milk or transplacentally, but transmission is more common from the mother's blood during delivery or during contact while caring for the baby.

198. *Idiopathic neonatal hepatitis* (a) comprises about 75% of neonatal

hepatitis; (b) is a familial disorder of autosomal recessive inheritance; (c) includes such histological features as the presence of giant
cells, focal necrosis, hemosiderosis, cholestasis, and loss of normal
zonal architecture; (d) may cause stillbirth or death during the
neonatal period or fluctuating jaundice during the first few months
of life; (e) has a mortality rate of about 25–30%, with cirrhosis
developing in about 20%; and (f) is treated symptomatically.

199. *Biliary atresia* (a) is defined as a congenital failure of development (atresia or hypoplasia) of a portion or all of the intrahepatic
and/or extrahepatic systems; (b) has as its dominating clinical feature cholestatic jaundice starting shortly after birth and persisting
thereafter; xanthomas may occur and biliary cirrhosis with signs
of portal hypertension develops within a few months; (c) is difficult
to distinguish from neonatal hepatitis—giant cells on liver histology
may be present in both; (d) is diagnosed with the help of liver and
biliary tract radionuclide scans (HIDA) that determine patency and
flow through the ducts; ultrasonography, which demonstrates the
absence of dilated ducts or the presence of abnormalities in their
size; and liver biopsy, which helps distinguish neonatal hepatitis
from biliary atresia; and (e) is managed depending on the distribution of the defect; in most cases, extrahepatic ducts are obliter-
ated and Kasai operation (hepatic portoenterostomy) should be
performed during the first months of life; rarely, the proximal bile
ducts are patent and surgical correction by Roux-en-Y jejunal anastomosis is possible; biliary atresia is one of the commonest indications for liver transplantation.

200. In *choledochal cyst* (a) the etiology is a congenital cystic dilatation of the common bile duct associated with narrowing at its
terminal portion; (b) most patients are asymptomatic, but others
may present with RUQ pain, obstructive jaundice, a RUQ mass,
or bile peritonitis as a result of rupture; (c) *cholangiocarcinoma* occurs
in about 3%; and (d) management is surgical, with most surgeons
removing the cystic dilatation and reconstructing the biliary tree.

201. *Caroli's disease* is a rare congenital malformation characterized by cystic dilatation of the intrahepatic bile ducts. Recurrent cholangitis is common and stones tend to accumulate in the dilated ducts. Treatment consists of antimicrobial agents for cholangitis and drainage of the common bile ducts to remove calculi.

202. *Congenital hepatic fibrosis* is an inherited (autosomal recessive) disorder characterized by dense fibrous bands containing bile ducts that surround normal liver lobules. Portal hypertension and associated renal defects (tubular ectasia and polycystic kidneys) are common. *Cholangiocarcinoma* or *hepatocellular carcinoma* are uncommon complications.

203. In *adult polycystic disease*, inheritance is dominant. Patients may be asymptomatic or may complain of abdominal pain, swelling, and pressure sensation, presenting during the fourth or fifth decade. Associated multiple renal cysts are very common (>50%), and the disease carries an excellent prognosis.

204. *Arteriohepatic dysplasia (Alagille syndrome)* is an autosomal dominant disorder characterized by chronic intrahepatic cholestasis presenting in the neonatal period and decreasing with age. Pulmonary stenosis, skeletal changes, and posterior embryotoxon are associated. Survival to adulthood is common but with physical and mental impairment.

205. *Reye's syndrome* is characterized by rapidly progressive encephalopathy with cerebral edema and fatty liver that develop a few days after a viral infection. Hyperammonemia, elevated SGOT levels, and hypoglycemia are common. An association with salicylate therapy has been suggested. Treatment is aimed at the relief of cerebral edema.

206. *Acute fatty liver of pregnancy* is an uncommon potentially fatal disorder characterized by acute liver failure occurring toward the end of a normal or "toxemic" pregnancy or shortly before or after delivery of a stillborn fetus. An association exists with IV administration of tetracyclines during pregnancy. Renal failure commonly accompanies liver failure. Mortality rate is around 75%, but the long-term prognosis of survivors is good.

207. *Hepatic granulomas* may be found on liver biopsy in sarcoidosis, tuberculosis, brucellosis, infectious mononucleosis, Hodgkin's disease, primary biliary cirrhosis, hypogammaglobulinemia and in a severe prolonged febrile syndrome of unknown etiology described by Simon and Wolff in 1973 (Simon WB & Wolff SM, Medicine (Baltimore) 52:1, 1973).

208. *Pyogenic liver abscess* may be caused (a) by obstruction of bile flow (by stones, tumor, sclerosing cholangitis, strictures); (b) by spread through portal blood flow (acute appendicitis, empyema of gallbladder, diverticulitis, perforated ulcer, pancreatitis); (c) by direct spread (trauma, perinephric abscess); or (d) idiopathically.

209. *Management of pyogenic liver abscess* includes antimicrobial agents (cefoxitin with an aminoglycoside or clindamycin with an aminoglycoside) combined with needle aspiration (the latter should be performed for large abscesses only). Surgical drainage is reserved for those patients who do not respond to these measures.

210. *Amebic abscess* (a) is usually solitary in the right lobe; (b) rarely has a history of amebic dysentery; (c) has as its main clinical features RUQ pain aggravated by change of posture and alcohol, with or without fever; (d) is diagnosed by the demonstration of a filling defect on radionuclide scan or ultrasonography, a positive amebic hemagglutination test, and the demonstration of amebic pus on needle aspiration; and (e) is treated with metronidazole, given orally 750 mg tid or intravenously 500 mg qid for 7–10 days; emetine, given intramuscularly in a dose of 1 mg/kg per day, is an alternative to metronidazole and is combined with the latter for 2–3 days in seriously ill or complicated cases.

211. In *schistosomiasis (bilharziasis)* (a) the liver may be infected by ova of *S. mansoni* or *S. japonicum* delivered from the intestine via the mesenteric veins; (b) the prevalence is high in the Far East, Africa, and parts of South America; (c) clinical features include hepatosplenomegaly followed by portal hypertension resulting from extensive liver fibrosis; hepatocellular function is relatively preserved, and the portal hypertension is presinusoidal; (d) treatment includes oxaminiquine or praziquantel; prevention is by avoidance of infected water; and (e) *hepatocellular carcinoma* is an occasional late complication.

212. *Etiological factors in primary hepatocellular carcinoma (HCC)* include (a) the mycotoxin aflatoxin (well documented), whose estimated ingestion (through contaminated food) parallels HCC incidence; (b) HBV, especially when infection occurs at an early age; HBsAg is produced by cell lines derived from human HCC; (c) alcohol (incriminated since HCC is more common in patients with alcoholic liver disease); (d) smoking (recently listed as a risk factor); and (e) rather frequently, advanced hemochromatosis.

213. *Clinical features of HCC* include (a) M:F ratio of 5:1; (b) associated cirrhosis (common); HCC should be excluded in any deterioration in the clinical course of a patient with cirrhosis; (c) RUQ pain and low-grade fever (common); (d) bleeding into the gut or intraperitoneally as a result of blood vessel erosion; (e) an arterial murmur due to increased vascularity or a friction rub due to perihepatitis (may occasionally be heard over the liver); (f) ascites (common), which may be aggravated by portal vein and/or hepatic vein thrombosis; and (g) hypercalcemia, hypoglycemia, hyperlipidemia, and polycythemia, probably reflecting ectopic hormonal production by the tumor.

214. *Alpha-fetoprotein* is commonly present in the serum of patients with HCC but is also found in the serum of patients with embryonic tumors of ovary and testis, hepatoblastoma, and liver metastases from carcinomas of the GI tract. Levels of 500 ng/ml are suggestive of HCC.

215. *Diagnosis of HCC* is suggested by the clinical features and elevated levels of alpha-fetoprotein. The tumor can be demonstrated by radionuclide scans, ultrasonography, and CT scan. There is a typical angiographic appearance.

216. In the *treatment of HCC* (a) if disease is confined to one lobe, resection is recommended; the presence of cirrhosis is a contraindication to an extensive resection; (b) chemotherapy (mainly adriamycin or combination chemotherapy) occasionally leads to symptomatic improvement or somewhat prolonged survival; (c) ligation of hepatic artery has been reported to have very limited success; (d) regional hepatic chemotherapy using an implantable drug infusion pump has met with limited success and many side effects; (e) radiotherapy is used for palliation of pain; and (f) results of liver transplantation for HCC are very disappointing, with tumor recurring after surgery; the only exceptions were small tumors discovered incidentally or HCC of the fibrolamellar type.

217. *Liver metastases* may be characterized as follows: (a) common (in 35–50% of all cancers); (b) common sites of the primary tumor are the organs with portal venous drainage, stomach, breast, and lung; (c) hepatomegaly is a common physical finding, and fever, pleuritic pain, and a friction rub over the liver may be present; (d) liver function studies (mainly alkaline phosphatase, bilirubin, and SGOT) may be abnormal, but normal values do not exclude the diagnosis; (e) ultrasonography and CT scan can demonstrate metastases, and needle liver biopsy will detect metastases, especially when they are distributed diffusely, with CT- or ultrasonography-guided biopsies increasing the yield; and (f) hepatic lobectomy for solitary metastasis is recommeded by many authorities but a definite prolongation of survival has yet to be documented.

218. *Liver transplantation* (a) is performed at many medical centers all over the world and is no longer an experimental procedure; (b) has as its potential candidate a patient with advanced irreversible liver disease who has become hospital bound; (c) is contraindicated in patients with psychiatric disorders, ongoing alcohol abuse, cardiopulmonary disease, extrahepatic malignancy, deep hepatic coma, and the presence of HBeAg in the serum; (d) has been indicated to date for nonalcoholic cirrhosis or CAH, biliary atresia in children, inborn errors of metabolism (alpha$_1$-antitrypsin deficiency, Wilson's disease, tyrosinosis, glycogen storage disease), hepatic malignancies, alcoholic cirrhosis (when prolonged abstinence was well documented), primary biliary cirrhosis, sclerosing cholangitis, and Budd–Chiari syndrome; limited experience has been accumulated in liver transplantation in acute liver failure (fulminant hepatitis and toxic hepatitis); (e) has shown improved survival when cyclosporin A was introduced as a part of antirejection therapy; overall 1-year survival is around 75% and is still improving each year; (f) demonstrates the best results in children with biliary atresia and in adults with relatively preserved hepatocellular function; (g) is associated with intra- and perioperative deaths due to hemorrhage and bile leakage, and these complications become uncommon as experience is gained; (h) has not been associated with hyperacute rejection to date, and acute rejection occurs mainly when immunosuppressive therapy is reduced or discontinued; chronic rejection manifests as chronic liver failure; rejection is diagnosed by repeated liver biopsies whenever a clinical or laboratory deterioration is observed and is treated by a course of high-dose antirejection chemotherapy; and (i) has become a promising therapeutic modality for end-stage liver disease.

Glossary

ARF	Acute renal failure
BAO	Basal acid output
BCAA	Branched-chain amino acids
BOG	Bacterial overgowth
BSP	Bromsulphalein
CAH	Chronic active hepatitis
CBD	Common bile duct
CCK	Cholecystokinin
CDA	Chenodeoxycholic acid
CEA	Carcinoembryonic antigen
CLH	Chronic lobular hepatitis
CMC	Critical micellar concentration
CPH	Chronic persistent hepatitis
CT	Computed tomography
DES	Diffuse esophageal spasm
DIC	Disseminated intravascular coagulation

DT	Delirium tremens
DU	Duodenal ulcer
ERCP	Endoscopic retrograde cholangiopancreatography
5-FU	5-Fluorouracil
GE	Gastroesophageal
GI	Gastrointestinal
GOT	Glutamic oxaloacetic transaminase
GPT	Glutamic pyruvic transaminase
GU	Gastric ulcer
HAV	Hepatitis A virus
Hb	Hemoglobin
HBcAg	Hepatitis B core antigen
HBeAg	Hepatitis B e antigen
HBsAg	Hepatitis B surface antigen
HBV	Hepatitis B virus
HCC	Hepatocellular carcinoma
Hct	Hematocrit
HDL	High-density lipoprotein
IBD	Inflammatory bowel disease
IBS	Irritable bowel syndrome
ICU	Intensive care unit
IF	Intrinsic factor
IM	Intramuscular(ly)
IMA	Inferior mesenteric artery
IV	Intravenous(ly)

IVC	Intravenous cholangiography
LDH	Lactic dehydrogenase
LDL	Low-density lipoprotein
LES	Lower esophageal sphincter
LLQ	Left lower quadrant
MAO	Maximal acid output
MCT	Medium-chain triglyceride
MEN	Multiple endocrine neoplasia (syndrome)
MMC	Migrating motor complex
NANB	Non-A–non-B hepatitis
N-G	Nasogastric (tube)
NMR	Nuclear magnetic resonance
NPO	Nothing per os
NSAID	Nonsteroidal antiinflammatory drugs
OCG	Oral cholecystography
PABA	p-Aminobenzoic acid
PAO	Peak acid output
PSE	Portal systemic encephalopathy
PT	Prothrombin time
PTC	Percutaneous transhepatic cholangiography
PTH	Parathyroid hormone
PTT	Partial thromboplastin time
PUD	Peptic ulcer disease
SBP	Spontaneous bacterial peritonitis

SMA	Superior mesenteric artery
TB	Tuberculosis
TPN	Total parenteral nutrition
UES	Upper esophageal sphincter
VIP	Vasoactive intestinal polypeptide
VLDL	Very-low-density lipoprotein
WHVP	Wedged hepatic venous pressure

Index

Citations are in the form chapter number:key fact number.